WR450

122

A Colour Atlas of the
Hair, Scalp and Nails

A Colour Atlas of the
Hair, Scalp and Nails

R. Baran MD
Head of the Dermatology Department
Centre Hospitalier
Cannes

R.P.R. Dawber MA, MB, ChB, FRCP
Consultant Dermatologist
Department of Dermatology
The Slade Hospital
Headington, Oxford

G.M. Levene MB, BS, FRCP
Consultant Dermatologist
Middlesex Hospital, and
St. John's Dermatology Centre,
St. Thomas's Hospital,
London

Wolfe Publishing Ltd

Copyright © R. Baran, R.P.R. Dawber, G.M. Levene, 1991
Published by Wolfe Publishing Ltd, 1991
Printed by BPCC Hazell Books Ltd, Aylesbury, England
ISBN 0 7234 0938 2

A CIP catalogue record for this book is available from the British Library.

This book is one of the titles in the series of Wolfe Medical Atlases, a series
that brings together the world's largest systematic published collection of
diagnostic colour photographs.

For a full list of Atlases in the series, plus forthcoming titles and details of
our surgical, dental and veterinary Atlases, please write to Wolfe
Publishing Ltd, 2–16 Torrington Place, London WC1E 7LT, England.

Contents

Preface

Every dermatologist and general practitioner sees a significant number of patients seeking help with disorders of the hair, scalp, and finger or toe nails. Diagnosis of these conditions is often far from straightforward since a wide variety of genetic, environmental, hormonal, cutaneous and systemic influences may be involved.

In this Atlas we illustrate the majority of common disorders, and some of the rarer ones, which affect these parts of the skin and its appendages. Attention is given to normal appearances, variations of normal with ageing, genetic disorders and the effects of environment, occupation and cosmetics. Important changes in the hair and nails which result from systemic disease are emphasized.

We believe that this Atlas will also be of value to chiropodists, cosmeticians and others dealing professionally with aspects of hair and nail care.

R. Baran
R.P.R. Dawber
G.M. Levene

Acknowledgements

Our collection of illustrations has been built up over many years. We wish to thank the many colleagues who have referred patients to us. We have acknowledged donors of illustrations in the text and we apologize if the names of others have been inadvertently omitted.

Introduction

Hair and nails are derived embryologically from the same tissue — the primitive epidermis (**1**).

In many skin disorders, hair and nail changes are commonly seen. Frequently, in acquired diseases that predominantly affect the epidermis, nail changes are present, while the hair follicles remain normal. The epidermis and nail apparatus grow continuously throughout life, while hair is produced intermittently in the hair cycle.

1

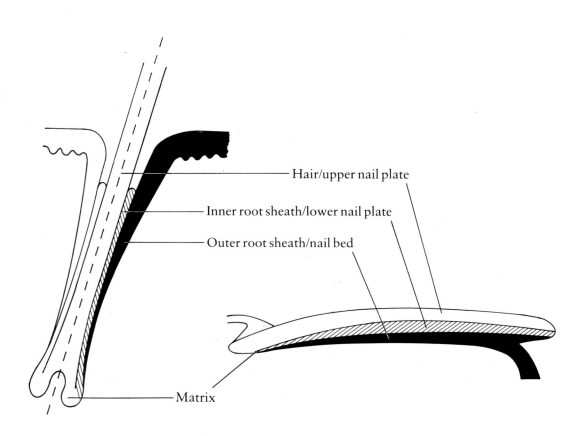

Hair/upper nail plate

Inner root sheath/lower nail plate

Outer root sheath/nail bed

Matrix

1 Similarity of hair and nail. (After·G. Achten.)

Hair

Introduction

Hair is not necessary to man for his survival, but it still has very important functions, and much anxiety and distress is generated when it becomes abnormal.

The functions of hair include:

- As an instrument of recognition, declaring identity. Hair distribution and style are important in individual and group image.
- Sexual attraction, by its appearance and as a carrier of apocrine secretion.
- As an important tactile organ: hair follicles have a liberal supply of fine nerve endings that respond to light touch.

In other primates and moulting animals, a coat of exact length and colour is seasonal and necessary for survival. The central medulla is also a heat conserver in certain species, e.g. the polar bear and the porcupine, in which medullary air spaces may take up more than 50% of the hair diameter. Moreover, the air spaces of the central medulla of many white and/or light-coloured animals enhance the whiteness (and thus the camouflage value) by increasing the amount of reflected light.

Note: even though most other primates are hairier than man, humans have more hair follicles per unit area of skin than other primates! Man thus has a greater potential for hairiness in response to an appropriate stimulus (such as hormones or drugs).

Hair embryology and development

Knowledge of the embryology of the hair follicle is desirable to enable one, first, to understand hair shaft structural abnormalities, and second, to appreciate that the sequence of hair formation in foetal life is partly recapitulated in each cycle of follicular activity.

The first human hair follicle rudiments appear at about 9 weeks *in utero* in those regions that in other animals bear tactile vibrissae — eyebrows, upper lip and chin. General hair development does not begin until the fourth month, with follicles developing in a cephalocaudal direction.

Each follicle is formed by local interaction between dermal and epidermal components. The first sign, or progerm, is a crowding of nuclei. The epidermal component grows downwards as a solid column of cells; ultimately its base envelops a papilla of dermis and becomes the matrix from which the hair and its associated inner root sheath develop. Initially, very fine lanugo hair forms.

In adults hair follicles are arranged in patterns, of which the group of three is the commonest. To form this pattern follicles first develop *in utero* at fixed intervals of between 274 and 350 μm; as the skin grows, new follicular rudiments grow between them when a critical distance has been reached. Normally, no new follicles develop after approximately 22 weeks *in utero*, although follicular density increases as the body surface increases. The main factors determining the amount of body hair are anagen and telogen duration, which vary greatly among individuals and from site to site in the same individual.

The first coat of long, fine lanugo hair is shed *in utero* between 32 and 36 weeks. Since growth of these hairs is synchronized, this shedding occurs rapidly as a moult. The second coat of shorter lanugo hair, in all areas except the scalp/eyebrows/eyelashes, where the hair may be longer and of larger bore, is also shed as a wave during the first 3 to 4 months of post-natal life; again, this occurs as a moult that may be almost imperceptible. The more or less unsynchronized mosaic pattern of hair growth then becomes established.

On the scalp *in utero* the hair is shed twice, apart from the occipital region, where only one shedding occurs; the delayed onset of telogen in this region results in the development of obvious occipital alopecia in some children during the early weeks of life. This delayed telogen may render the hairs more prone to frictional damage. Complete recovery is the rule.

The area of the scalp destined to develop mature coarse, long and pigmented hair is often called the scalp hair field; the boundaries of this field separating it from areas producing only very fine short hair may be abnormally placed anteriorly or posteriorly in various rare genetic syndromes.

2

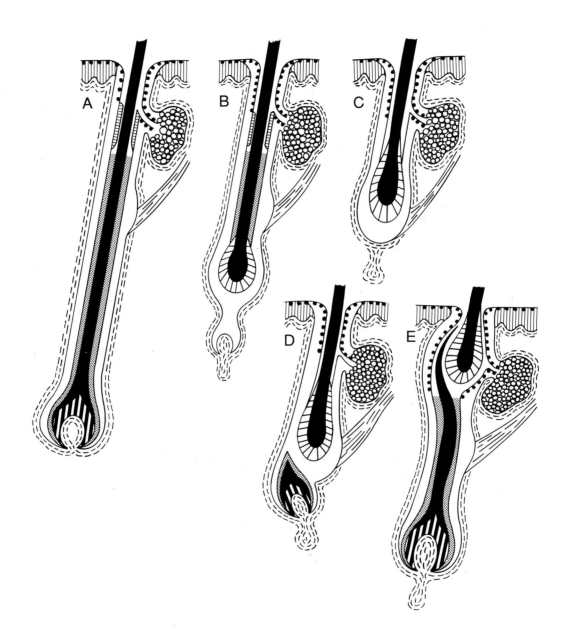

2 Phases of the hair cycle. A, mature anagen (metanagen); B, catagen; C, telogen; D, early anagen; E, later anagen phase showing new hair growing in the same connective tissue sheath, eventually displacing the previous hair, which is shed.

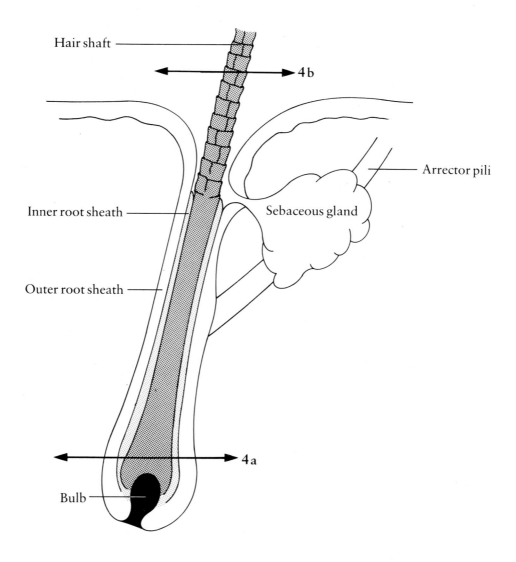

Hair shaft

4b

Arrector pili

Inner root sheath

Sebaceous gland

Outer root sheath

4a

Bulb

3 Vertical section diagram of mature hair. Arrowed lines show levels of transverse sections shown in **4a** and **4b**.

Linear hair growth. Scalp hair, approximately 1 mm every 3 days (1 cm per month). Growth shows much individual variation, but is more or less constant from childhood to old age. The figures given here are from a Japanese study.

Site variations

Vertex	0.44 mm/day
Chest	0.44 mm/day
Temples	0.29 mm/day
Beard	0.27 mm/day

Follicular structure

The mature growing (anagen) follicle has the structure shown in **4**. It consists of six ascending concentric rings of cells, all differentiating from a single stem cell population, the hair matrix; only the inner three layers will produce the central hair shaft — the medulla, cortex and cuticle of the definitive hair shaft. The outer root sheath (ORS) is a sleeve of epidermis overlying the inner root sheath (IRS); it is essentially of the same structure as, and is continuous with, the interfollicular epidermis of the scalp.

The exact function of the root sheaths is not known, although they are intimately related to the developing hair layers. The IRS hardens before the hair within it does, so that it plays an important part in defining the shape and diameter of the hair.

Hair colour is essentially governed by the amount of melanin pigment in the hair. This is derived from melanocytes intimately associated with the bulb matrix cells, which donate pigment granules to those cells that become the hair cortex (7). The actual colour depends on the type of melanin deposited, but the various shades of colour are due to the size, shape, distribution and density of melanin granules within the hair cortex.

4a

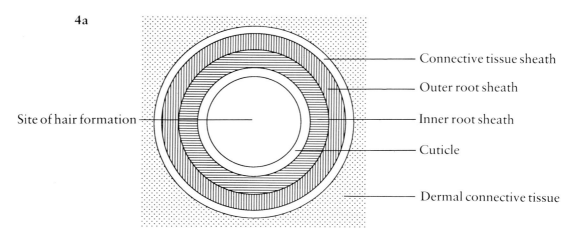

Site of hair formation

Connective tissue sheath

Outer root sheath

Inner root sheath

Cuticle

Dermal connective tissue

4a Cross section of hair follicle.

4b

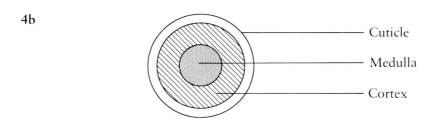

Cuticle

Medulla

Cortex

4b Cross section of individual hair.

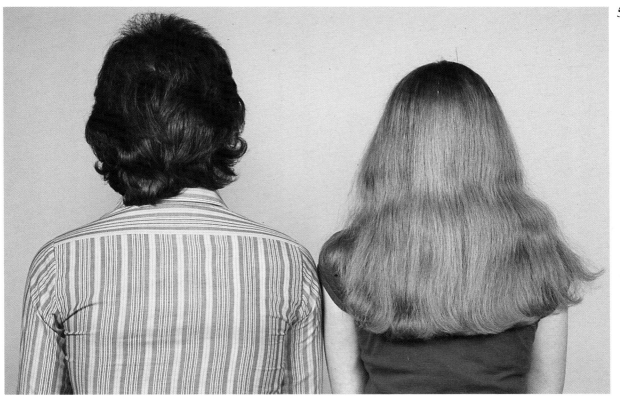

5 **Comparative length of hair that has not been cut for more than 6 months in a 24-year-old male (left) and a 27-year-old female (right).** The longer hair in the female is due to the longer anagen phase in women. This may be even longer during pregnancy when telogen shedding may be minimal.

Dynamics of follicular activity.

Anagen length: approximately 2 to 5 years
Catagen length: approximately 35 days
Telogen length: approximately 100 to 150 days

Total number of scalp follicles: approximately 100,000

Follicle density: newborn: 1135/cm^2
1 year: 795/cm^2
15 years: 615/cm^2

Highest anagen/telogen ratio is in childhood (scalp): more than 95%.

Scalp hair diameter:
- Rapid increase up to approximately 4 years of age.
- Slow increase from 4 to 10 years of age.
- Little further increase up to puberty.

6

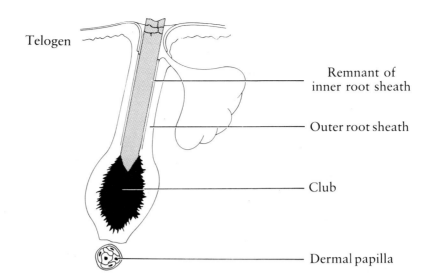

Telogen

Remnant of
inner root sheath

Outer root sheath

Club

Dermal papilla

6 Vertical section diagram of telogen hair showing 'club' morphology.

7

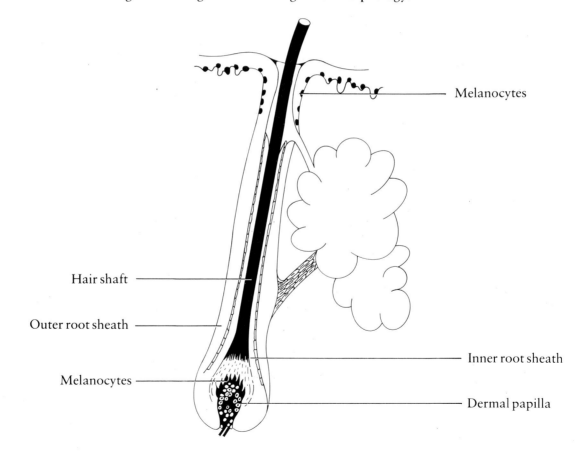

Melanocytes

Hair shaft

Outer root sheath

Melanocytes

Inner root sheath

Dermal papilla

7 **Source of hair pigmentation (vertical section diagram).** Melanocytes are present at the apex of the dermal papilla and donate pigment via melanosomes to the hair matrix cells, which subsequently differentiate to form the hair cortex.

Hair shaft structure

The definitive, hardened, hair shaft is basically composed of compacted, mostly longitudinally oriented, keratinized cells; its bulk is in the cortex. In man the central medulla may be continuously present, intermittent or absent in coarse, long, pigmented hairs — i.e. terminal hairs; it is absent in the short, hypo- or apigmented vellus hairs that cover most of the body in post-natal life, and also from the long, intra-uterine lanugo hairs.

The outer layers of flattened, overlapping cuticular cells (like roof tiles), which are very rich in dense, high sulphur protein, are well adapted (normally) to withstand environmental, chemical and physical forces tending to cause hair degeneration. Despite this, orderly breakdown of the hair shaft, particularly on the scalp, does occur: the process of weathering. Microscopically, such changes are usually only obvious in the distal 2–3 cm of hair that is longer than approximately 15 cm. They consist of fragmentation and loss of cuticular cells, fissures in the cuticle layer, and exposure and separation of cortical cells; some long hairs normally show terminal fraying, due to exposure of the long, fusiform cortical cells (see **17**).

Most books show the definitive hair as a long, cylindrical structure of circular bore. Scalp hair bore, however, varies with race: mongoloid hair is generally circular in cross section and straight; negroid hair is oval and tightly curled or crimped; while caucasoid hair varies, but is most typically slightly ovoid and wavy. Negroid hair is thought to weather more easily than other racial types because, first, its oval structure is more liable to friction degeneration, and second, it is thought to contain cortical areas of less dense keratin.

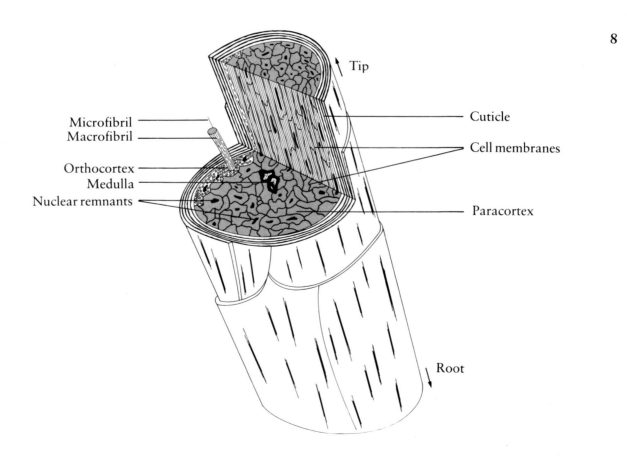

8 Ultrastructure of hair shaft.

Hair cycle

Unlike the epidermis and nail matrix, which divide continuously throughout life, the hair follicle only produces hair intermittently, going through a cycle of growth (the anagen phase), shrinkage (catagen phase) and rest (telogen phase), during which, certainly on the scalp, it is shed. The transition phase from growth to rest is known as the stage of involution. Depending on age, site, race, hormones and many other factors, the duration of each phase varies. On the scalp, anagen lasts approximately 5 years for each follicle, catagen about 5 weeks, and telogen about 5 months. These figures are for areas without evidence of significant common baldness. With increasing age and some scalp disorders the anagen phase shortens, leading to increased daily shedding of hair and a shorter maximum length of hair.

Linear hair growth is more or less maximal at all times, whatever the body site. Therefore the length to which hair will grow depends on the length of the anagen phase, rather than on variation in any theoretical speed of growth.

During the resting phase, the dermal papilla, which is thought to orchestrate the hair matrix and consequently the hair cycle and hair growth, does not disappear, but contracts into a ball of apparently inert cells underlying the telogen (club) root. The mechanism by which the dermal papilla reactivates and stimulates new follicular growth is not known. In humans, removal of the papilla generally prevents follicular growth; transplanted dermal papillae can produce new follicle formation from the overlying epidermis. The matrix cells that grow during the new anagen phase may form from the outer root sheath cells.

On the normal scalp, 80% to 95% of follicles on the vertex are in anagen phase. This is assessed by telogen counts, i.e. root microscopic analysis of plucked hairs, which may show up to 15% telogen roots in normal individuals. Occipital telogen counts are consistently lower after puberty in all age groups: typically less than 12%. Since under normal circumstances telogen hairs are shed, out of a population on the scalp of approximately 100,000 follicles, 100 to 150 hairs may be lost a day (after puberty). The fact that scalp hair follicles traverse the hair cycle out of synchrony with their neighbours means that moulting does not occur, and also that a careful status quo is maintained — in health, scalp hair volume and density remain largely unchanged.

With increasing age beyond puberty, the major factor changing scalp hair is common baldness on the vertex in both sexes; on other body sites, in the absence of illness hair in general changes little until the fifth or sixth decade, when in all areas some slight thinning of hair develops.

Hair cycle control/endocrine factors

Individual follicles appear to be under the control of the dermal papilla associated with each hair bulb. After puberty the main controlling influences on hair growth are hormonal. The major hormonal influence occurs when androgen production develops at puberty. Terminal hair replaces vellus hair, first in the pubic region, then in the axillae and subsequently over forearms, abdomen, buttocks, chest, back, arms and shoulders. The transition from vellus to terminal hair on the face also occurs in an orderly sequence: corners of the upper lip, then chin, cheeks, and on the rest of the beard area. The full pattern of terminal hair production does not reach its maximum extent until the fifth or sixth decade. The degree of vellus-to-terminal hair transformation described above is dependent on complex genetic and racial factors, mediated by androgenetic stimulation in both sexes.

It is paradoxical that the same androgenetic stimuli that convert vellus to terminal hair on the sites mentioned above promote terminal hair regression to secondary vellus hair on the vertex from puberty onwards. However, in the first few months of life, the influence of maternal androgens may lead to frontal patterning with bitemporal recession of a type that may recur after puberty. The degree of post-pubertal vellus regression on the vertex — common baldness (androgenetic alopecia) — also depends on complex racial and genetic factors in both sexes. Why normal men commonly produce patterned common baldness but women of the same genetic strain only develop diffuse thinning remains unclear, but it is likely to be a difference in follicular receptivity and reactivity to androgens, limited in some way by oestrogens. For example, after the menopause, when oestrogen production decreases, more androgenetic activity may be seen: increased vertical thinning and mild hirsutism, particularly on the lower face, this being entirely physiological.

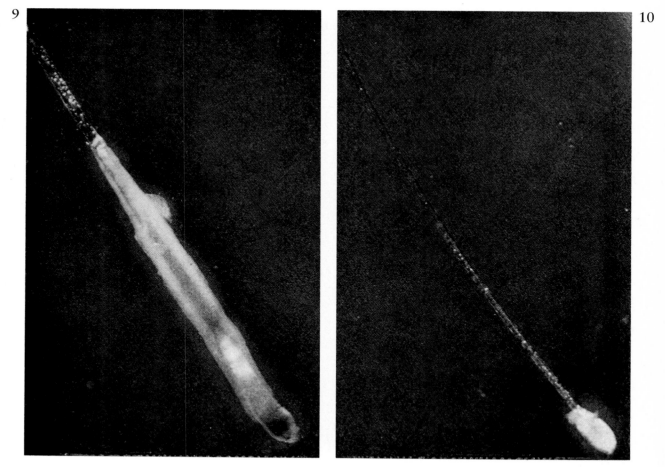

9, 10 **Normal plucked hairs (scalp).** Fully mature anagen (A) and telogen 'club' (B) roots (light micrograph).

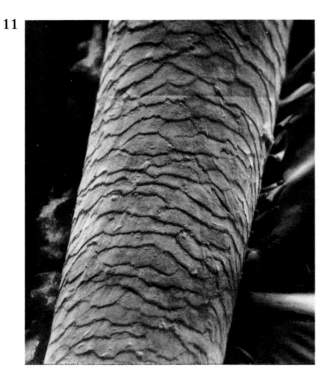

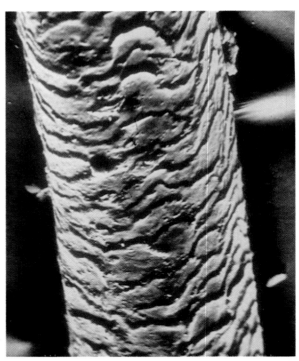

11 Normal hair, root end with unweathered, closely apposed, overlapping cuticular scales. (Scanning EM.)

12 Normal hair, appearances more distal to 11. Cuticular scales are raised and show breakage at their free margins (scanning EM).

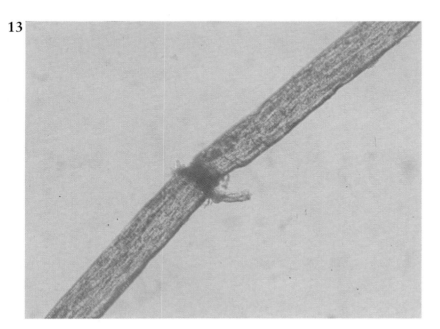

13 Weathering of hair, showing irregular hair shaft bore, loss of cuticular cells and a transverse fissure leading to an early node of trichorrhexis nodosa (light micrograph).

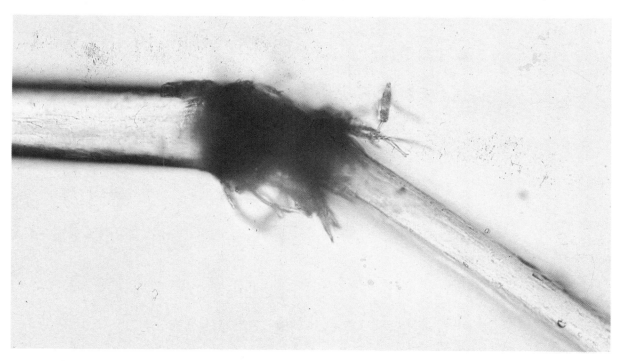

14 Weathering of hair, trichorrhexis nodosa type lesions. Such nodes may occur on normal long or negroid hair, in syndromes with increased congenital or hereditary hair fragility, and due to hair cosmetic abuse (e.g. excessive permanent waving, straightening and bleaching) (light micrograph).

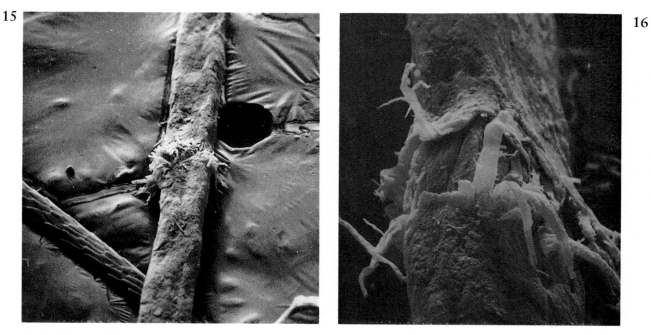

15, 16 Normal hair, same weathering changes as in **13** and **14** shown by scanning EM.

17

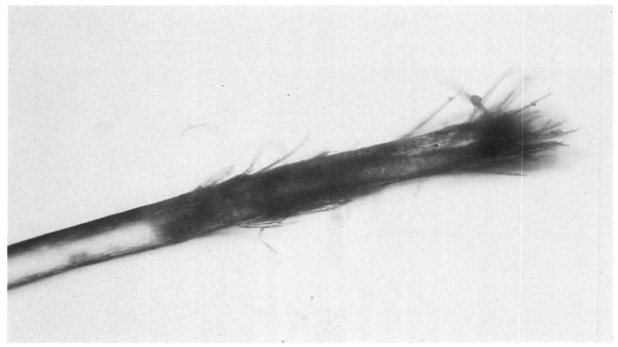

17 Weathering of hair: brush tip; changes typically seen in conjunction with those of **14** (light micrograph).

18

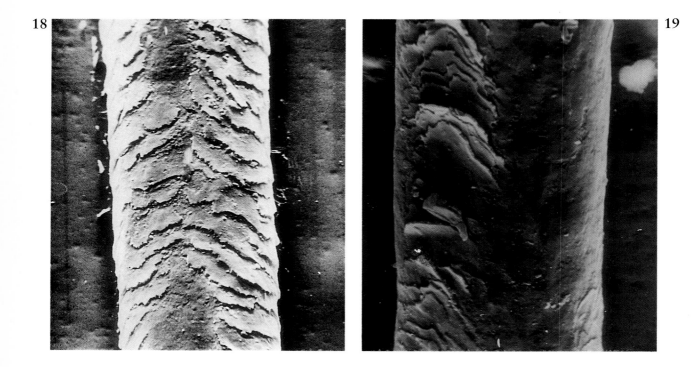

19

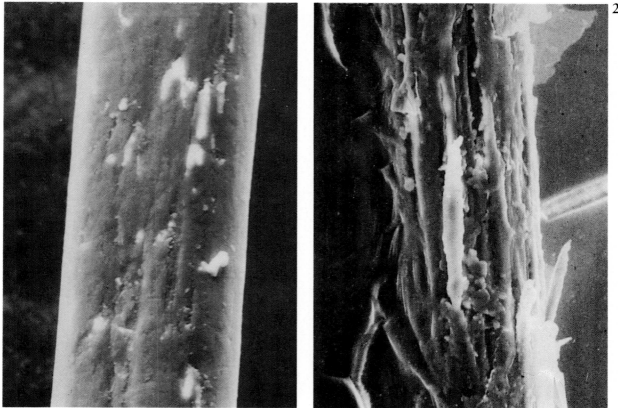

18–21 Normal hair, progressive cuticle loss, fissuring and exposure of cortical cells. In normal hair these changes are usually seen near the tip. In congenitally fragile hair, such as occurs in trichothiodystrophy, and hair that has undergone excessive cosmetic treatment, the changes may occur more proximally along the shafts (scanning EM).

22

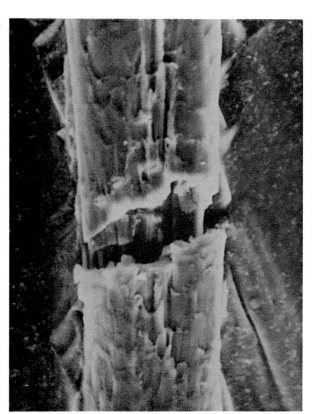

22 **Weathering of hair**, same stage as in **13**. (Scanning EM.)

23

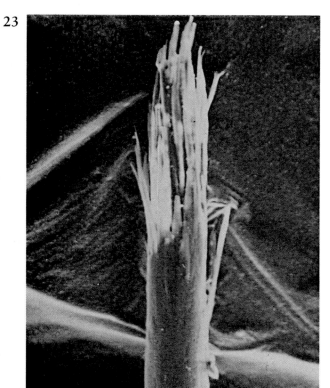

23 **Normal weathered hair**, same stage as in **17**. (Scanning EM.)

Hair disorders in infancy and childhood

Some hair disorders are manifest at or soon after birth. A few of these are shown in this section. Others are shown under the appropriate specific heading.

- Occipital alopecia of the newborn.
- Congenital alopecia.
- Aplasia cutis.
- Congenital focal hypotrichosis.
- Idiopathic hypotrichosis.
- Focal lumbo-sacral hypotrichosis.

- Congenital hypertrichosis lanuginosa.

There are a considerable number of genetic congenital ectodermal dysplasias in which there is sparse hair. By definition there is a diffuse epidermal abnormality, present from birth, which also affects at least one other appendage, especially the hair or nails. They are often associated with mental retardation, and skeletal, dental and other abnormalities.

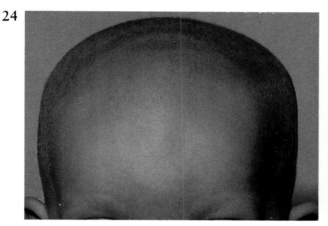

24 Congenital alopecia: total absence of hair from birth. Most examples are sporadic, but autosomal dominant inheritance occasionally occurs.

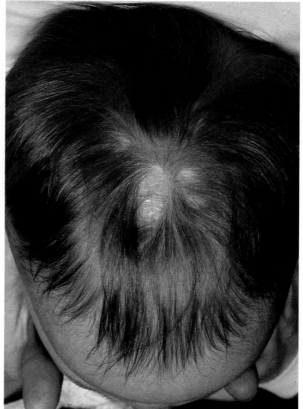

25 Aplasia cutis, scarred patch on the central vertex region. Such patches are present from birth either as an ulcerated area that heals by scarring, or as a patch simply without hair. Hereditary (autosomal dominant) and sporadic cases occur; rarely, other defects may be associated, e.g. anomalous veins, cerebral atrophy, spastic paralysis and mental retardation.

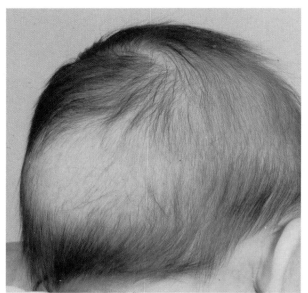

26 Congenital alopecia of the newborn.

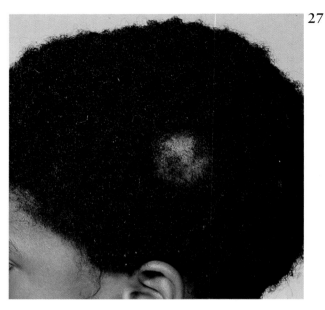

27 Congenital focal hypotrichosis: no scarring occurs in such areas.

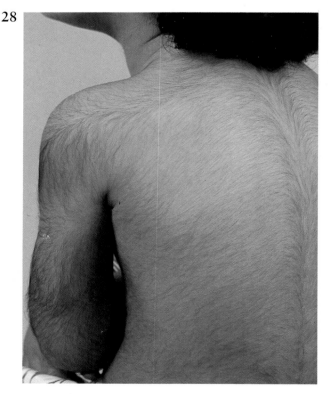

28 Idiopathic hypertrichosis. This degree of hypertrichosis may be seen as a normal racial phenomenon in certain Mediterranean or Asian groups, or as a cryptogenic change in any racial type with no other associated defects.

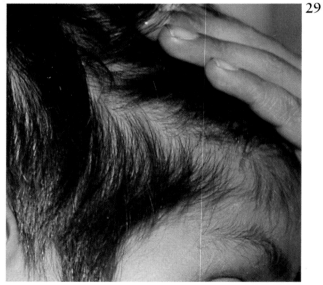

29 Normal low frontal and temporal hair line with hypertrichosis in an Asian (Indian) child. No androgen-related abnormalities are associated with this type of hairiness, which is present from early childhood when the first obvious terminal hair develops.

30 Focal lumbo-sacral hypertrichosis (faun tail). This tuft of long silky hair probably consists of retained lanugo hair. It is present at birth and persists throughout life. It may be associated with underlying spinal dysraphism and spinal cord or cauda equina damage with neurological impairment. Such changes, most common in early childhood, may be delayed for several years.

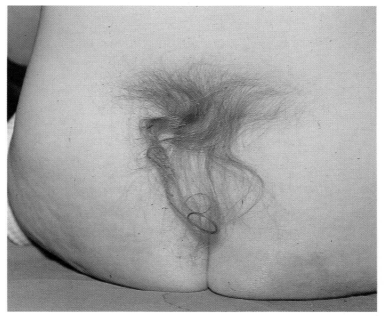

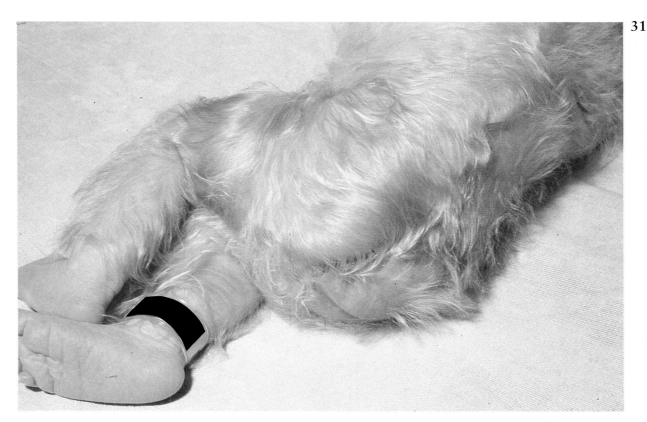

31 Congenital hypertrichosis lanuginosa (hypertrichosis universalis congenita). Inheritance is by an autosomal dominant trait, variable penetrance; rarely autosomal recessive. Most cases show the excessive hair from birth or develop such hair from the second to the seventh year, this type often resembling idiopathic hypertrichosis (**28**). (Courtesy Dr. J. Partridge.)

Physiological androgenetic alopecia (common baldness).

Progressive patterned thinning of scalp hair is seen in all populations and is normally more obvious in men than in women. Hairs change from the long thick pigmented terminal form to the fine pale vellus form (secondary vellus hair formation). The age of onset and rate of progression of this process is very variable.

Two main forms, Hamilton and Ludwig, are recognized, and are graded according to severity.

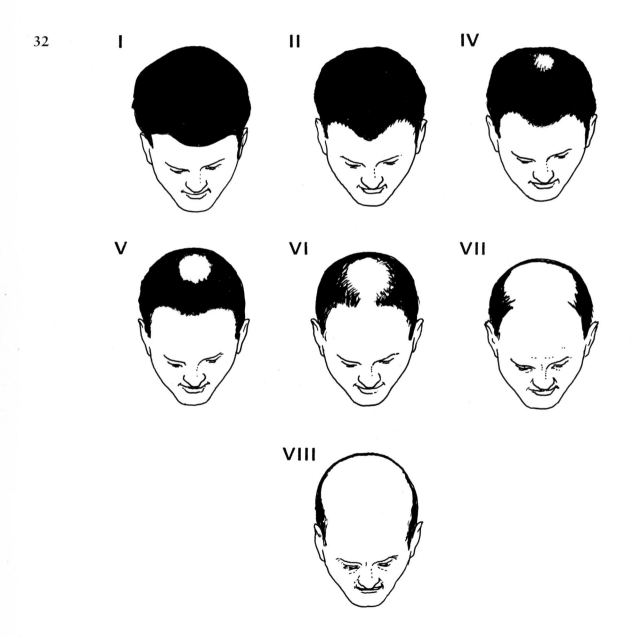

32 Hamilton's classification of scalp hair distribution (1951).

33 Androgenetic alopecia: Hamilton grade II in a man.

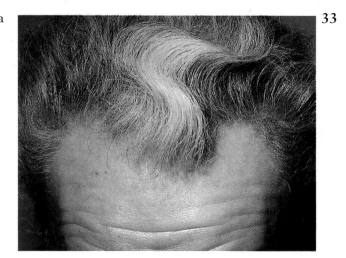

34 Androgenetic alopecia: Hamilton grade II/III in a man.

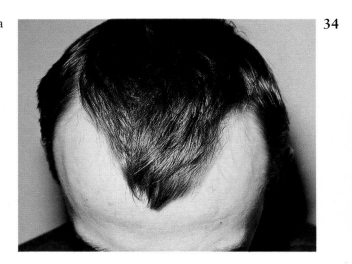

35 Androgenetic alopecia: Hamilton grade IV in a man.

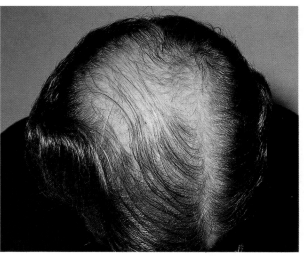

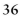

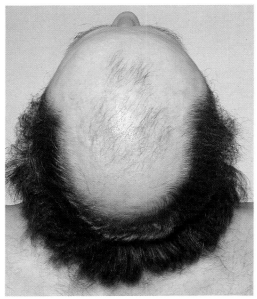

36 Androgenetic alopecia: Hamilton grade VIII in a man.

37 Scalp hair of Hamilton grade I in a woman: commonest pattern in both sexes before puberty, but in only a proportion of females after puberty.

38 Frontal hair lines and stylistically raised hair style as seen in photographic models. This Hamilton grade I pattern is suggested as normal in fashion magazines.

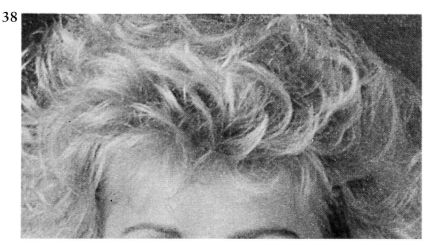

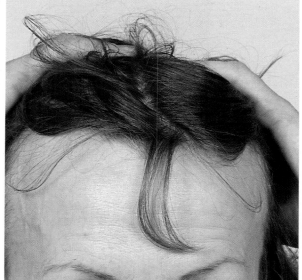

39 Hamilton grade II in a woman.

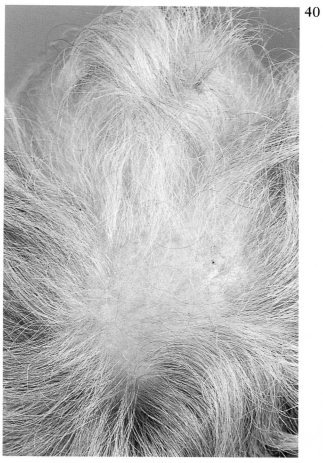

40 Hamilton grade IV in a woman.

41 Hamilton grade V in a woman.

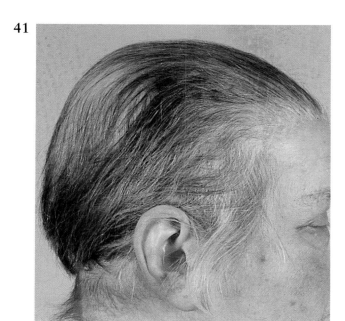

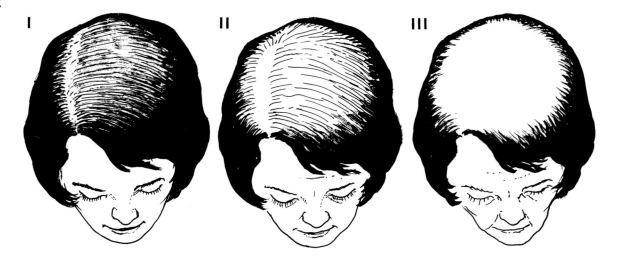

42 Ludwig's classification of scalp hair distribution in females.

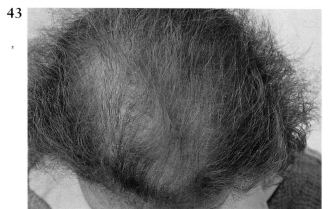

43 **Androgenetic alopecia (female):** Ludwig grade I. Note preserved frontal hair line.

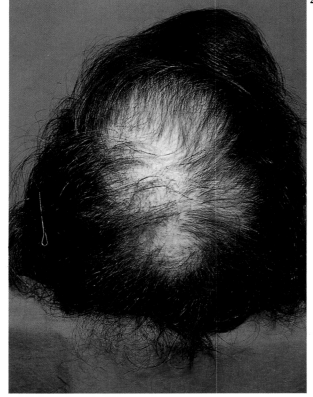

44 **Androgenetic alopecia (female):** Ludwig grade II.

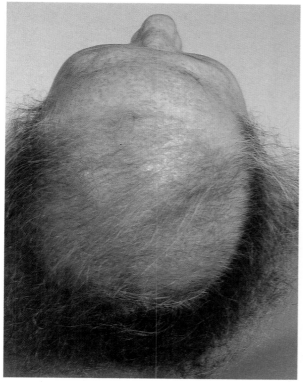

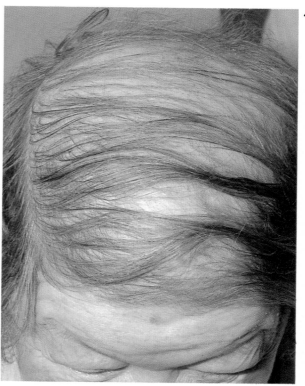

45 Androgenetic alopecia (female): Ludwig grade III.

46 Androgenetic alopecia (female): Ludwig grade III.

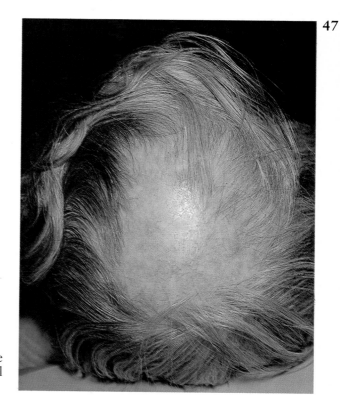

47 Androgenetic alopecia (female): Ludwig grade III with severe hair loss but retention of the frontal hair line.

Hirsutism

By hirsutism is meant the growth of terminal hair in those areas influenced by androgens to produce secondary sexual hair growth in the male: i.e. beard, moustache, chest, lower abdomen, back and limbs. Individual, genetic and racial variation is very great, and there is no clear distinction between physiological and pathological hirsutism. It is a problem complained of mainly by women in the potentially reproductive years, and is sometimes associated with high androgen levels and scanty or abnormal periods. After the menopause a degree of hirsutism is very common.

Hirsutism is to be distinguished from hypertrichosis, which is terminal hair growth appearing inappropriately and for reasons other than the influence of androgens.

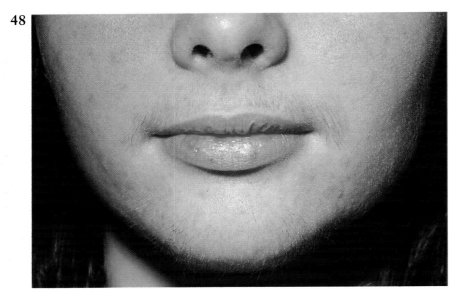

48 Facial hirsutism; idiopathic type on lower face in a 24-year-old woman. Slight acne vulgaris is also seen.

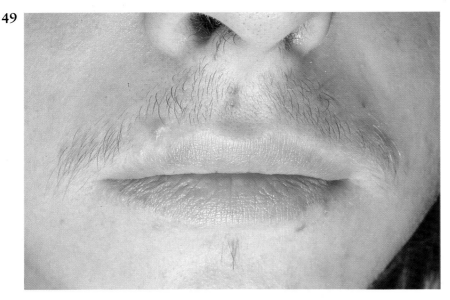

49 Hirsutism: moustache area in a woman. Inflamed follicular papules result from electrolysis treatment.

50 Hirsutism: jaw line and neck.

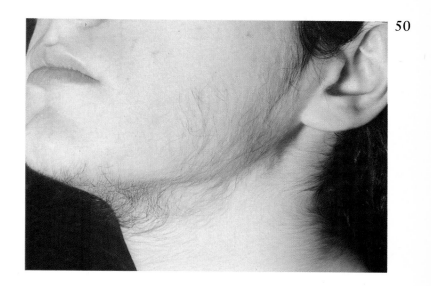

51 Hirsutism: chin and jaw line.

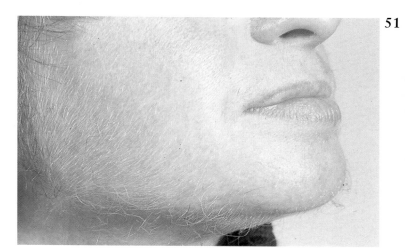

52 Post-menopausal hirsutism.

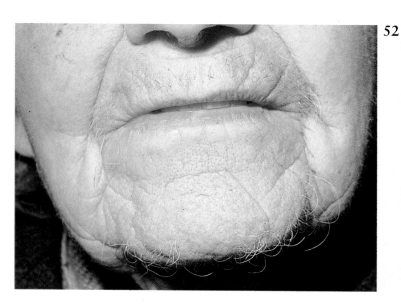

53

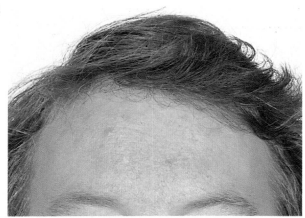

53, 54 Normal androgenized adult female with shaved chin, seborrhoea, slight acne and slight frontal hair recession. In these patients with facial hirsutism varying manifestations of virilism and hyperandrogenism may be associated, although hormone levels in the blood and urine will mostly be within normal limits on testing.

54

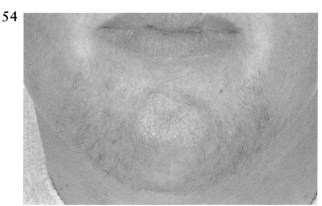

55 Hirsutism, some degree of unacceptable coarse hair growth, needing cosmetic removal, occurs in up to 10% of women at some stage after puberty. Other signs of possible virilism must always be looked for in this type of patient, but most are cryptogenic.

55

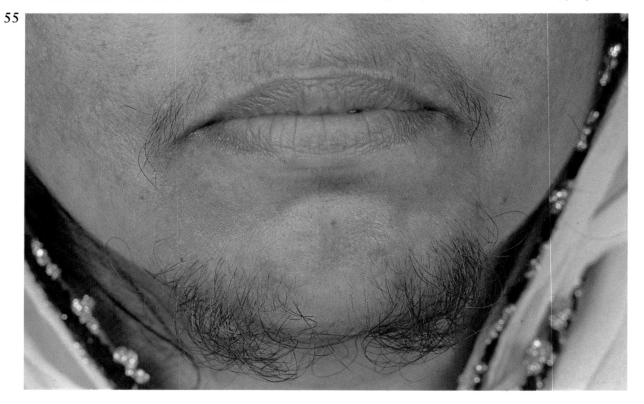

Diffuse alopecia

Diffuse alopecia is common following pregnancy. Otherwise it may be caused by external (physical) factors, by systemic disorders, by drugs, and, rarely, by genetic disorders.

The physical factors are:

- Trichotillomania, the accepted (if not very satisfactory) term used for compulsive pulling out of hair by the patient. Scalp, eyebrows, eyelashes or other hair may be affected.
- Scratching due to inflammatory scalp disease.

- Excessive cosmetic manipulation, massage, traction, hot and cold combing.

The systemic disorders are:

- Post-febrile (**166**).
- Hypothyroidism.
- Anaemia (iron deficiency).
- Cytotoxic drugs.
- Diffuse type of alopecia areata.
- Secondary syphilis (**163**).

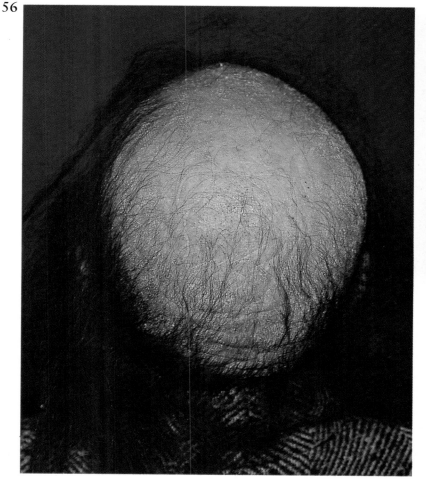

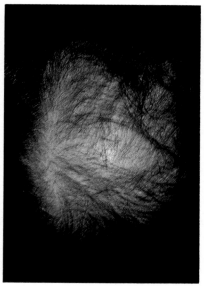

57 **Drug alopecia.** Diffuse (sometimes complete) alopecia is common during therapy with cytotoxic drugs; there is usually complete regrowth after the drug is stopped. Other drugs known to cause hair loss in some patients are heparinoid and coumarin anticoagulants, antithyroid drugs, vitamin A in excessive doses, and systemic retinoids. Thallium salts cause hair loss as a toxic effect.

56 **Hypothyroidism, if gross, can cause severe diffuse alopecia.** Related dry skin and mild cutis verticis gyrata are also evident in this patient.

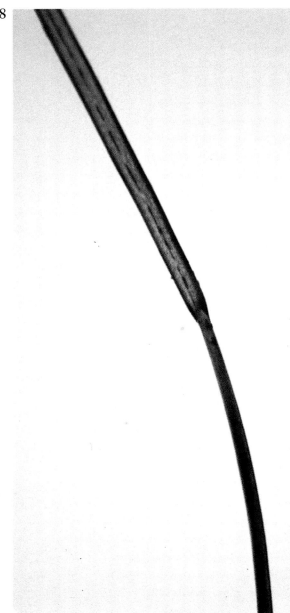

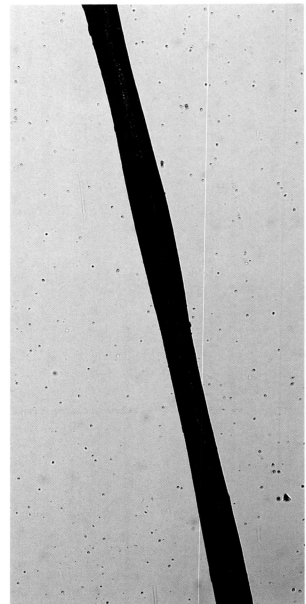

58 Narrowing of the hair shaft due to cytotoxic drug therapy that did not cause shedding, i.e. no anagen effluvium. Hair may break at the narrow section.

59 Monilethrix-like intermittent narrowing of the hair shaft due to bolus doses of cytotoxic drug therapy without anagen effluvium. Similar changes can be caused by illness (the Pohl–Pinkus constriction).

Structural defects of the hair shaft

Structural defects of the hair shaft with increased fragility include:

- Monilethrix.
- (Pseudomonilethrix).
- Pili torti.
- Netherton's syndrome (bamboo hair).
- Trichorrhexis nodosa.

Structural defects of the shaft without increased fragility include:

- Pili annulati (ringed hair).
- Woolly hair.
- Woolly hair naevus.
- Uncombable hair syndrome (*cheveux incoiffables*).

- Straight hair naevus.

Other abnormalities of the shaft are:

- Trichoptilosis (splitting of ends of hair shaft caused by physical and chemical trauma, see **17**).
- Pohl–Pinkus constriction (hair shaft narrowing due to illness or a drug, see **59**).
- Trichonodosis (knotting of hair).
- Trichostasis spinulosa (retention of telogen hairs in large pilo-sebaceous follicles).
- Weathering of hair shaft (see **15, 16, 19–23**).

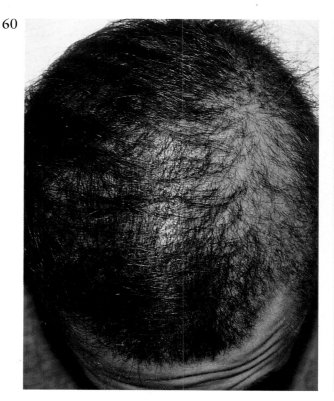

60 Monilethrix, showing short, broken scalp hairs of irregular length. The hairs are beaded and brittle (see **63**).

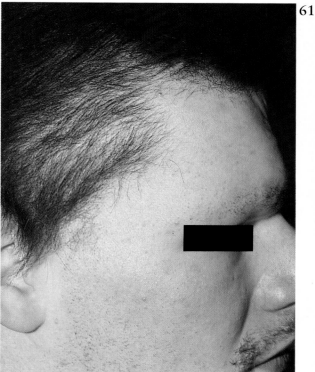

61 Monilethrix: longer, less weathered and broken hair than in **59**; the eyebrows are also affected in this case.

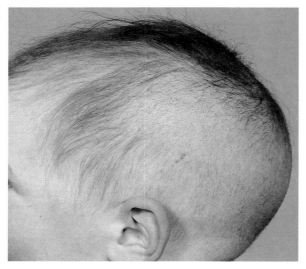

62 Monilethrix: severe, irregular hair loss in a young child.

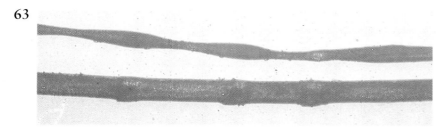

63 Monilethrix (lower hair) and pseudomonilethrix (upper hair), light micrograph. Pseudomonilethrix is an artefactual condition produced in microscopic mounting by hairs pressed across each other. Monilethrix shows clear beading.

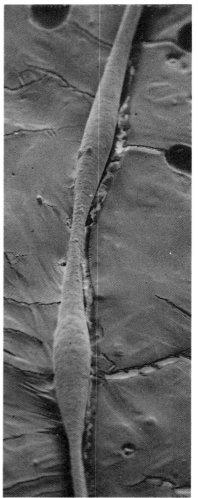

64 Monilethrix (EM).

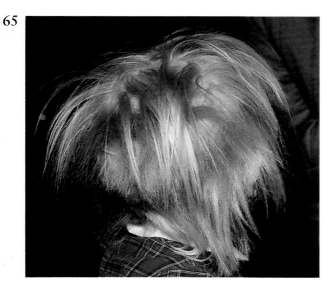

65 Pili torti. The classical unruly hair of this condition is shown, associated with irregular breakages and weathering of hair.

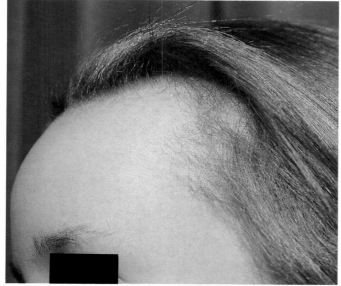

66 Pili torti: longer, less weathered hair than in the case in **65**. Affected hairs have a spangled appearance in reflected light.

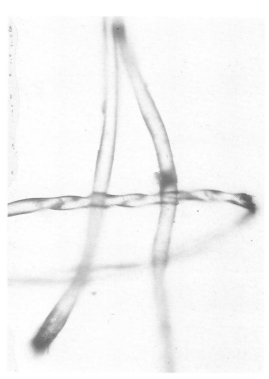

67 Pili torti: low power light micrograph showing many 180-degree twists and some trichorrhexis nodosa-type weathering.

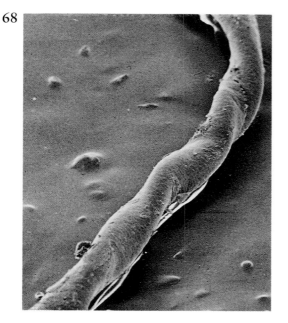

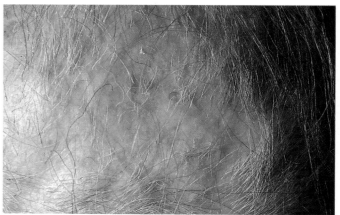

68 Pili torti: scanning EM showing twisted hair shaft. This section shows very little weathering, the surface cuticular scales being normal.

69 Pili torti: acquired focal irregular type commonly seen in progressive scarring alopecias where scarring within the follicle (prior to complete follicular disappearance) interferes with normal hair keratinization and hardening.

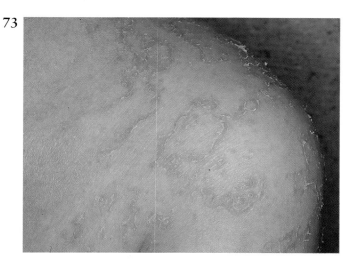

70 Netherton's syndrome. The scalp hair is dry and brittle and patchily sparse. Erythema and scaling of the face are visible. (Courtesy Dr W.A. Branford.)

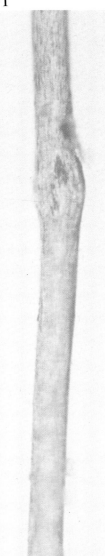

72 Netherton's syndrome. Same case as in **71** showing bamboo nodes with some degree of invagination within the nodes (trichorrhexis invaginata).

71 Netherton's syndrome: low power light micrograph showing bamboo cane-type nodes. The hair in this condition may weather badly and show associated trichorrhexis nodosa-type changes.

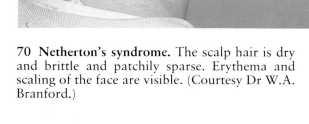

73 Netherton's syndrome: skin lesions. The skin is dry and shows variable patterned inflammatory lesions (known as ichthyosis linearis circumflexa). (Courtesy Dr W.A.D. Griffiths.)

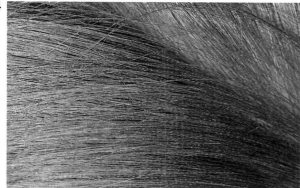

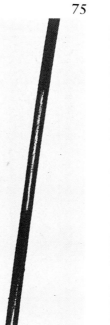

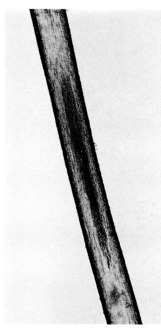

74 **Pili annulati** (**ringed hair**), showing alternating light (abnormal) and dark bands along each hair shaft. Usually inherited as an autosomal dominant trait.

75 **Pili annulati:** low power light micrograph, showing two dark abnormal bands with a normal pale central area.

76 **Pili annulati:** light micrograph, transmitted light showing a dark central band.

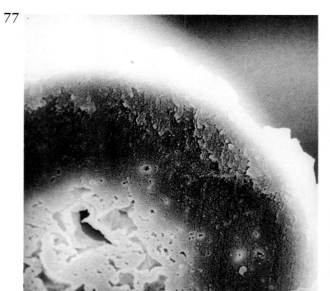

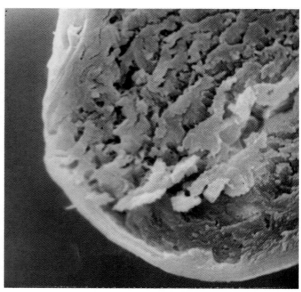

77 **Pili annulati:** scanning EM transverse section through a normal band showing outer ring of dense compact hair cortex with fenestrated central medulla.

78 **Pili annulati,** scanning EM. Transverse section through an abnormal band showing the pathological basis of the condition: diffuse irregular spaces throughout the cortex.

79

80

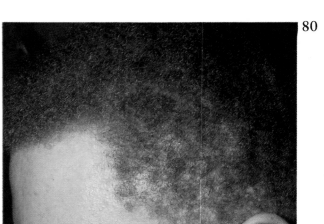

79 Woolly hair: congenital or hereditary wool-type crimping and curling of hair of the whole scalp. Most cases are sporadic.

80 Woolly hair: hereditary or congenital type affecting the whole scalp.

81

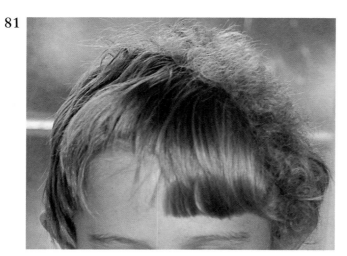

81 Woolly hair naevus. A focal equivalent of **79**. This type may inherit varying types of epidermal naevus in association.

82

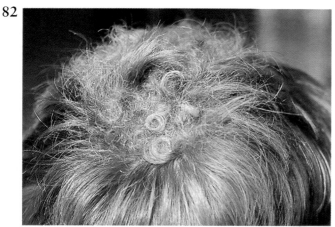

82 Woolly hair naevus.

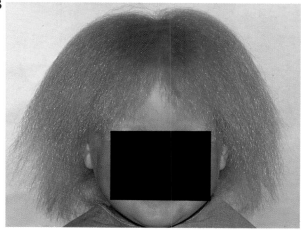

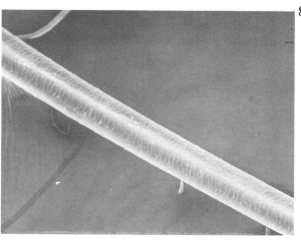

83 *Cheveux incoiffables*. (Synonyms: spun glass hair, pili trianguli et caniculi, uncombable hair syndrome.) This abnormality is fixed and obvious from birth, or when the first terminal hair grows during the first year of life. It remains unchanged throughout life. (Courtesy, Department of Dermatology, Royal Victoria Infirmary, Newcastle upon Tyne.)

84 *Cheveux incoiffables*. Showing a canalicular gutter along the hair shaft. (Scanning EM.)

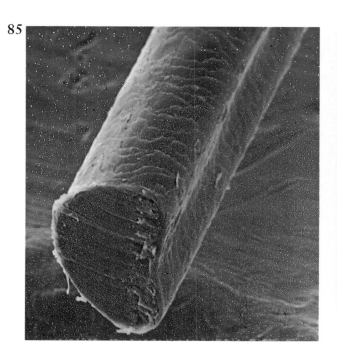

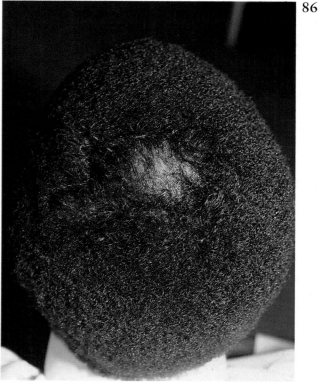

85 *Cheveux incoiffables*. Showing the roughly triangular cross section of the hair shaft. (Scanning EM.)

86 Straight hair naevus, a focal naevus in which fixed uncurly hair is seen in negroid subjects.

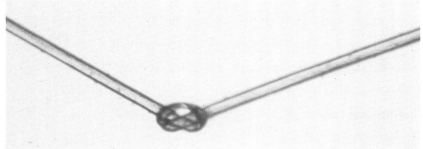

87 Knotting of hair. Synonym: trichonodosis. This cosmetically originating abnormality is relatively common in negroid subjects and caucasoids with curly hair. The knots occur spontaneously during cosmetic procedures such as combing and brushing (light micrograph).

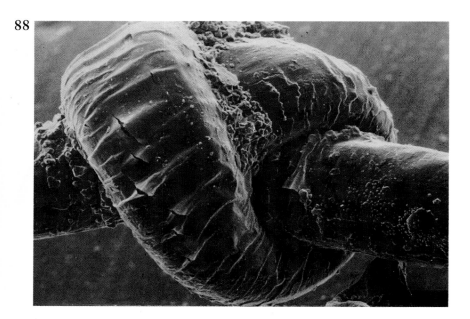

88 Knotting of hair, scanning EM showing cuticular fissures due to the knot.

Hypertrichosis

Hypertrichosis is growth of hair excessive for the site and the age of the patient, specifically excluding androgen induced hirsutism.

- Congenital hypertrichosis lanuginosa (see **31**).
- Idiopathic hypertrichosis.
- Congenital circumscribed hypertrichosis:
  (a) associated with congenital melanocytic naevi.
  (b) Becker's naevus.
  (c) lumbo-sacral hypertrichosis (see **30**).
  (d) naevoid hypertrichosis.
- Acquired hypertrichosis lanuginosa (this rare condition in adults, more in women than in men, is usually associated with an internal carcinoma).
- Drug induced hypertrichosis.

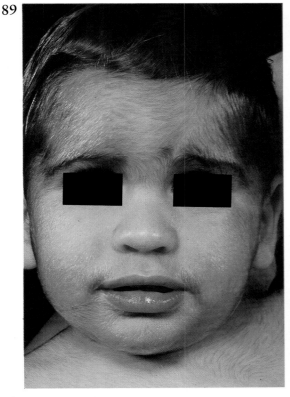

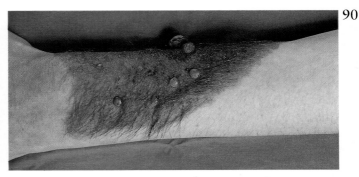

90 Hairy pigmented congenital melanocytic naevus.

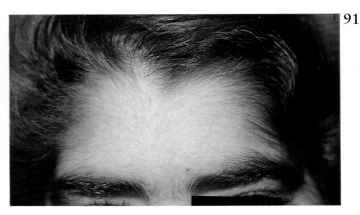

89 Idiopathic hypertrichosis. Note the small terminal hairs on the forehead, bushy eyebrows and prominent eyelashes. This type of hypertrichosis can occur in all races. Such changes may be an isolated sign in otherwise normal children; severest forms may be part of a variety of syndromes, e.g. Cornelia de Lange syndrome.

91 Drug induced hypertrichosis, following administration of oral minoxidil for malignant hypertension. About four out of five patients so treated develop obvious hypertrichosis requiring regular cosmetic treatment.

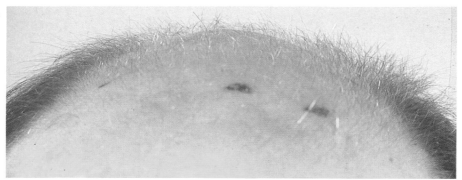

92 Drug induced hypertrichosis, after taking diazoxide for hypertension. Hypertrichosis using this drug is less severe than that caused by minoxodil.

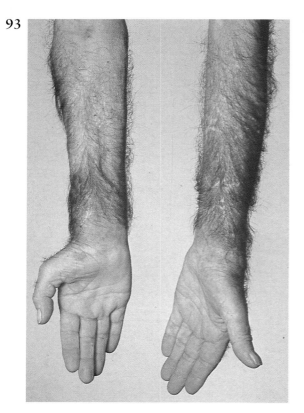

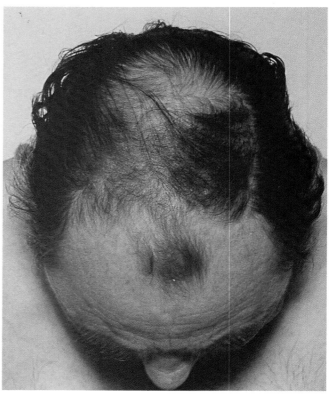

93 Drug induced hypertrichosis, due to cyclosporin-A immunosuppressive treatment following organ transplantation. None of the coarse hair seen on the forearms was present prior to the drug therapy. This degree of hypertrichosis is unusual with this drug.

94 Drug induced hypertrichosis caused by cyclosporin-A. There is considerable fine regrowth of hair on the previously bald scalp. (Same patient as in 93.)

Traumatic alopecia

- Cosmetic traumatic alopecia, resulting from use of excessive or inappropriate cosmetic procedures, leading to physical or chemical damage to the hair.
- Trichotillomania, pulling out of hair by the patient as part of a psychological disturbance.
- Accidental traumatic alopecia (due to accidental trauma).

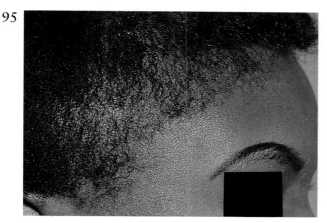

95 Traumatic alopecia, showing diffuse hair loss due to a combination of traction and straightening with a hot comb.

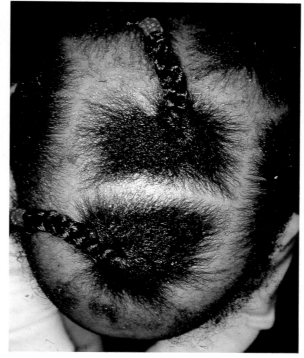

96 Traction alopecia: loss of hair at margins of the plaited areas. (Courtesy Dr. J. Leonard.)

97 Patchy occipital hair loss in a child, in this case due to a traction hair style and associated friction and pressure.

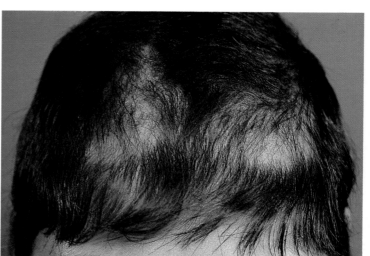

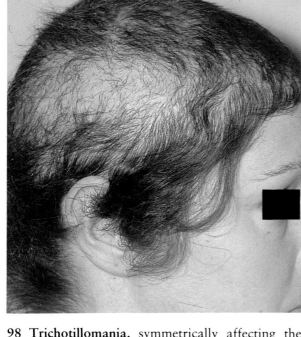

98 Trichotillomania, symmetrically affecting the vertex. Known as the tonsure type. The pattern almost exclusively affects adult, unmarried women.

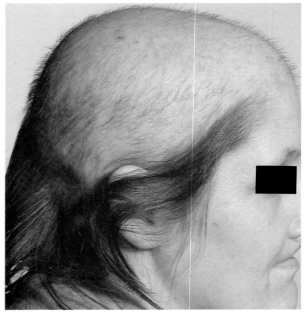

99 Trichotillomania: small localized patch in a child. It usually returns to normal within 1 to 2 years. It has no significant associated psychological problem, and is itself no more significant than temporary childhood nail biting.

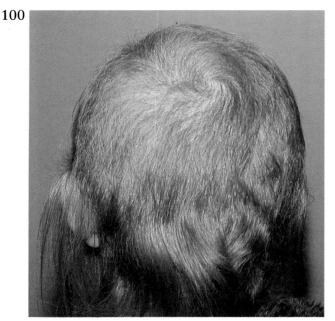

100 Tonsure trichotillomania: rear view showing the typical sign of retention of long normal hair in the occipital marginal area.

101 Tonsure trichotillomania: severe case with very short hair in the affected areas.

102 Tonsure trichotillomania: subtle hair loss mimicking Ludwig type of androgenetic alopecia.

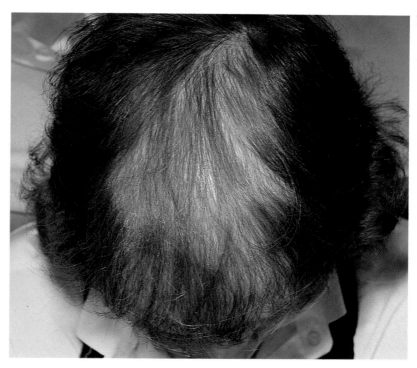

103 Tonsure trichotillomania: severe type showing the even length of short hair in the affected area.

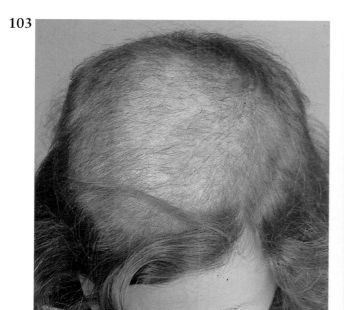

104 Trichotillomania: sharply marginated tonsure type, with a poor prognosis. This followed unequivocal alopecia areata, trichotillomania being a rare sequela.

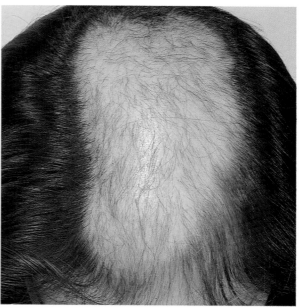

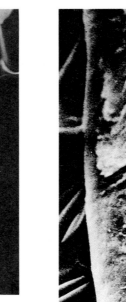

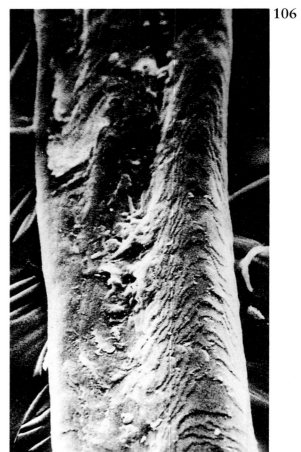

105, 106 Acute hair damage seen after immersion in permanent wave or hair straightening solutions (scanning EMs).

Alopecia areata

Alopecia areata is a condition of unknown cause that starts with patches of baldness on the scalp, or elsewhere, in childhood, adolescence, or in adult life. Patches usually regrow, but in a minority of patients the condition spreads to produce total scalp alopecia or universal alopecia. There is sometimes a family history of the condition, or of autoimmune disease. An increased incidence occurs in diabetes mellitus, autoimmune thyroid disease, vitiligo, pernicious anaemia and Addison's disease. Alopecia areata occurring in association with atopic disorders (atopic dermatitis, or asthma) or Down's syndrome is likely to be severe. In some patients psychological stress appears to precipitate attacks.

Nail changes in the form of pitting are found in some cases of acute and chronic alopecia areata (see 357, 358).

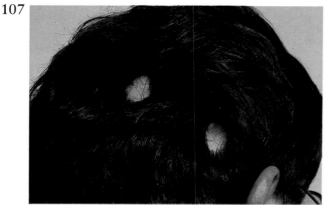

107 **Alopecia areata:** two isolated lesions within the scalp. This type, occurring in isolation, has the best prognosis.

108 **Alopecia areata,** reticulate patchy variety. This pattern usually precedes the development of alopecia totalis or universalis.

109 **Alopecia areata,** reticulate patchy variety.

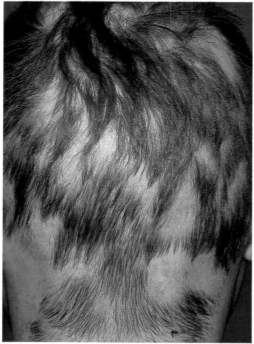

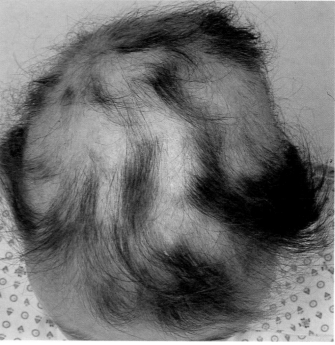

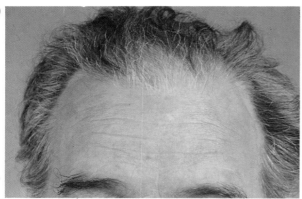 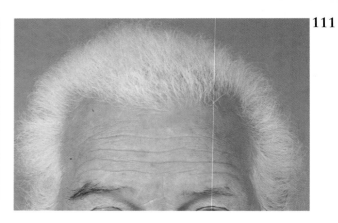

110, 111 Apparent rapid onset of grey hair, occurring within days; due to alopecia areata preferentially affecting pigmented hairs.

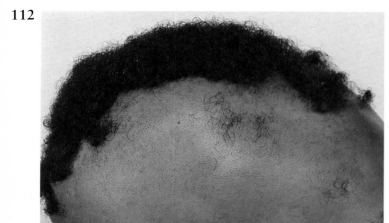

112 Alopecia areata: severe marginal (ophiasis) form which has spread around the scalp. This type has a poor prognosis for regrowth.

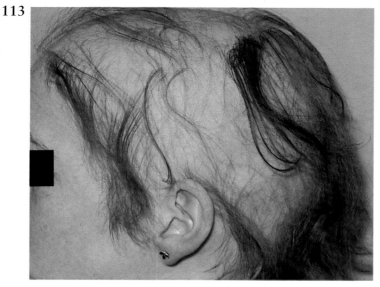

113 Alopecia areata, diffuse, acute shedding type: usually rapidly progresses to alopecia totalis or universalis.

114 Alopecia areata: loss of right eyebrow and partial loss of eyelashes.

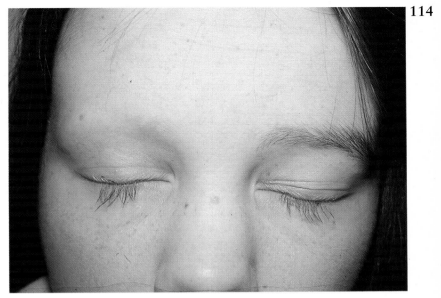

115 Alopecia areata of the forearm.

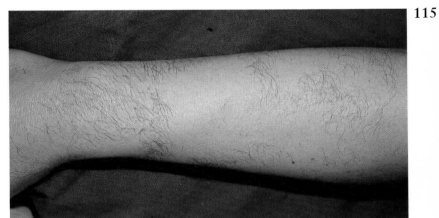

116 Alopecia areata: a single presternal patch.

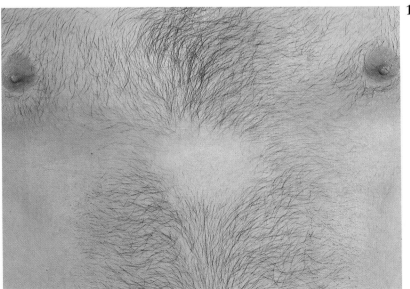

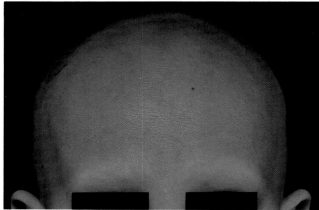

117 Alopecia areata: alopecia totalis, with loss of eyebrows and eyelashes.

118 Alopecia areata: exclamation mark hairs. At the margins of active lesions are often found small hairs that are of normal width at the tip and narrow at the base, giving the appearance of an exclamation mark. They are pathognomonic in alopecia areata.

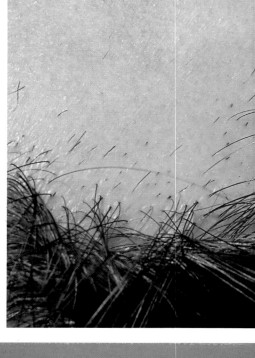

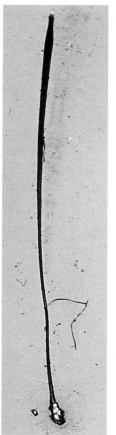

119 Alopecia areata: a plucked exclamation mark hair showing the telogen (club) root, a narrow section above, and distally a wider pigmented section with a fractured tip.

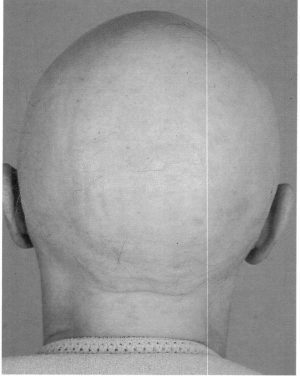

120 Alopecia areata: alopecia totalis variety involving the whole scalp. This pattern has a poor prognosis for regrowth.

121 Alopecia areata, showing patchy loss of hair from the beard area in a dark shaven individual. This may be misdiagnosed as vitiligo because of the pallor due to hair loss.

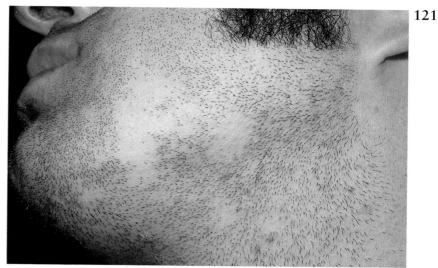

122 Alopecia areata: unpigmented regrowing hair on the scalp.

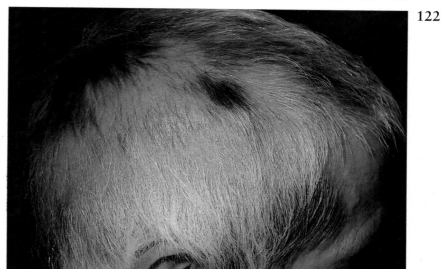

123 Alopecia areata: hypopigmented regrowing hair after alopecia totalis.

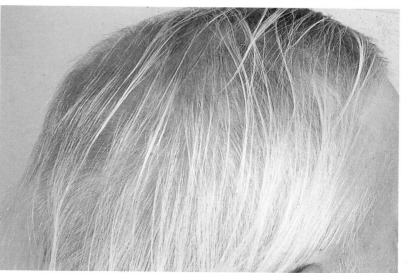

Cicatricial alopecia

In cicatricial alopecia there is destruction of hair follicles and often damage to the interfollicular skin. Diagnosis is often difficult and biopsy of the margin of the affected area is usually necessary, but even histology is not always diagnostic.

The more important forms of scarring alopecia are:

- Pseudopelade.
- Folliculitis decalvans.
- Lichen planus (pilaris).
- Lupus erythematosus (see **198, 199, 200, 201**).
- Cicatricial pemphigoid (see **206**).
- Erosive pustular dermatosis of the scalp.
- Cicatricial alopecia from physical trauma.
- Chronic radiodermatitis.
- Localized scleroderma.

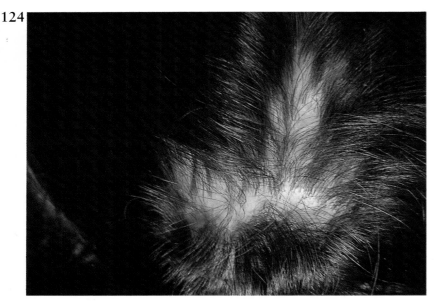

124 Pseudopelade: progressive follicular loss without inflammation, of unknown cause. Skin biopsy is necessary to exclude inflammatory disease.

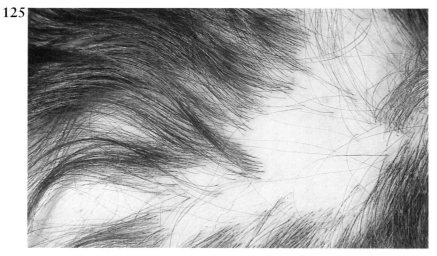

125 Pseudopelade: a more severe example.

126 Folliculitis decalvans, showing areas of follicular pustulation. This spreads irregularly, leaving behind patchy follicular scarring.

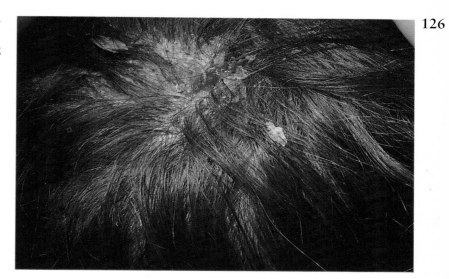

127 Scarring alopecia, folliculitis decalvans type, showing central scarring and spreading peripheral crusting and pustulation due to pus-forming organisms, usually staphylococci.

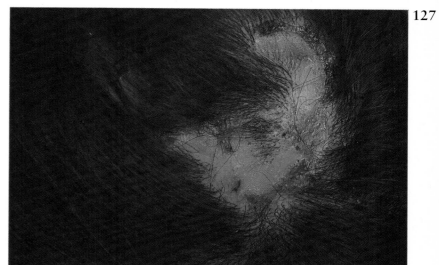

128 Folliculitis decalvans, showing follicular pustulation.

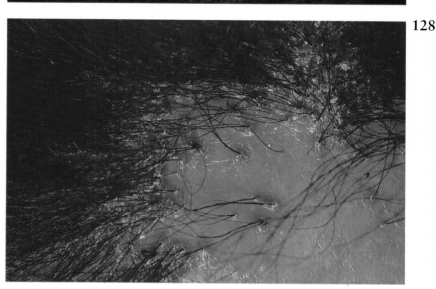

129

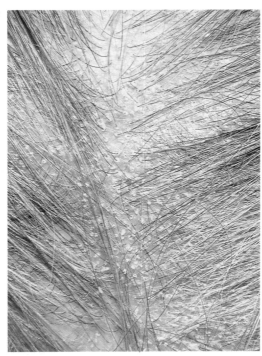

129 Lichen plano-pilaris: the form of lichen planus that attacks hair follicles and can cause rapid and permanent loss of scalp hair. More typical lichen planus lesions are often, but not always, present elsewhere on the skin.

130

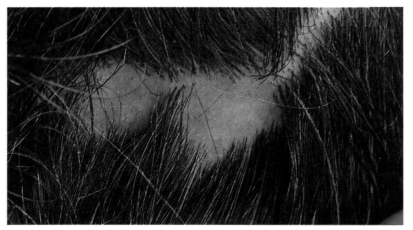

130 Lichen planus: two patches on the scalp showing dull red follicular inflammation spreading outwards and leaving scarring in its wake. Clinical signs in this type are not entirely diagnostic, and histology is necessary.

131

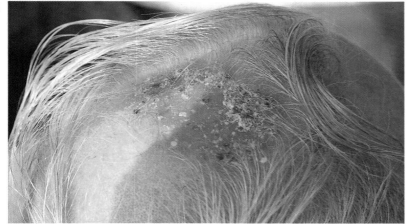

131 Erosive pustular dermatosis of the scalp, showing crusted, pustular lesions. This is classically a condition of old age, often precipitated by minor trauma, particularly in sun damaged skin.

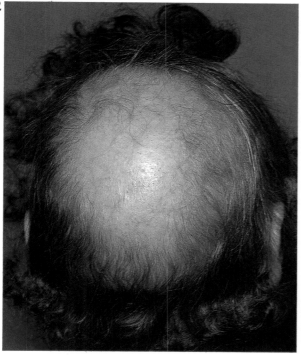

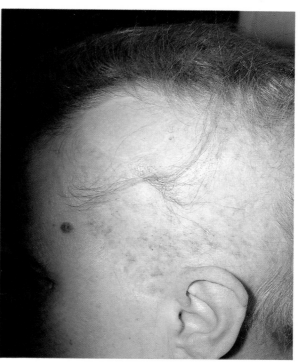

132 Diffuse scarring (cicatricial) alopecia, due to X-ray epilation for childhood tinea capitis 30 years previously.

133 X-ray alopecia resulting from radiation treatment of childhood scalp ringworm. Malignant tumours (basal and squamous cell carcinomas) commonly arise in X-ray damaged skin many years after irradiation, and a skin graft shows where such a tumour was removed.

134 Localized scleroderma (morphoea) of the frontal scalp region: the so-called *en coup de sabre* appearance. Such lesions may be associated with underlying bone atrophy; in childhood, facial hemiatrophy of bony structures is sometimes seen.

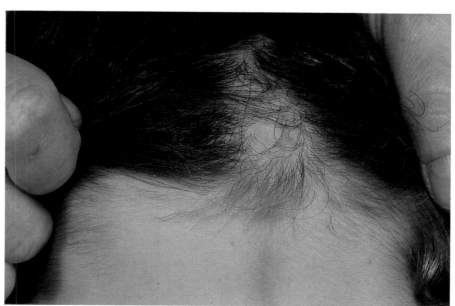

134

Hair colour

Normal hair colour is under genetic control and the four common colours are black, brown, red and blond. Genetic variation is seen with many intermediate normal colours. Scalp hair tends to darken with age, before it turns grey or white. Various types of melanin account for hair colour.

People with red hair have pale skin that tends to burn easily in the sun and to show poor resistance to skin irritants.

Normal and abnormal variations in hair colour include:

- Blonde hair.
- Normal greying of hair.
- Premature greying of hair.
- Vitiligo.
- Poliosis (localized patches of white hair due to deficient melanin in a group of adjacent follicles).
- Hereditary defects.
- Albinism.
- Colour changes induced by drugs and chemicals.
- Colour changes due to nutritional deficiencies.

135

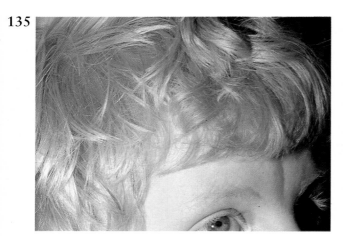

136

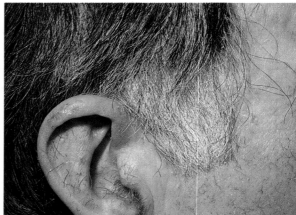

135 Blond, blue-eyed individual. This youth is normal; this colouring is associated with a higher than average incidence of: (a) phenylketonuria; (b) vitiligo; (c) gluten enteropathy; and (d) pernicious anaemia.

136 **Normal greying of hair,** particularly obvious on the sideburns.

137

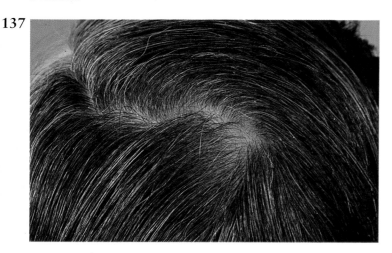

137 **Normal middle aged greying of hair;** also shows a normal clockwise whorl on the crown.

138 Early or premature greying of hair. This normal phenomenon is significantly associated with pernicious anaemia, vitiligo, and some other disorders associated with autoimmune antibodies.

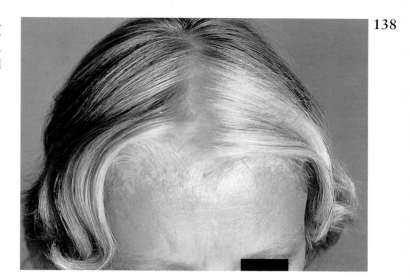

139 Vitiligo: patchy, sharply marginated depigmented lesions are seen at the scalp margin and on the face and neck. They deceptively resemble areas where hair has fallen out.

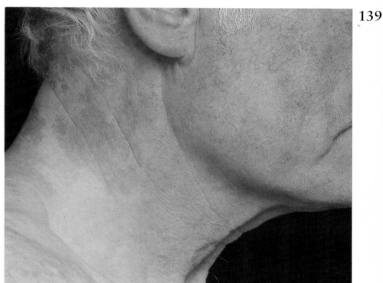

140 Vitiligo, affecting pigmentation in a lock of scalp hair; no hair loss occurs.

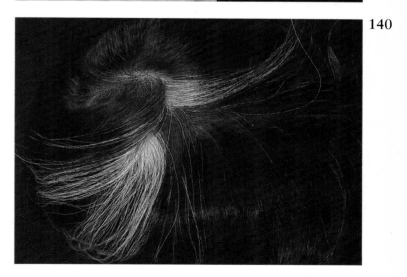

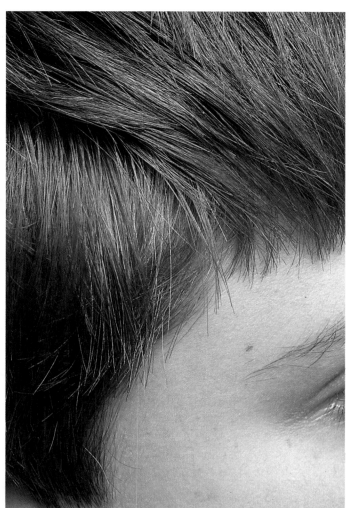

141 Vitiligo, showing a few hair shafts with pigment loss; but at no stage is hair lost (see also alopecia areata).

142

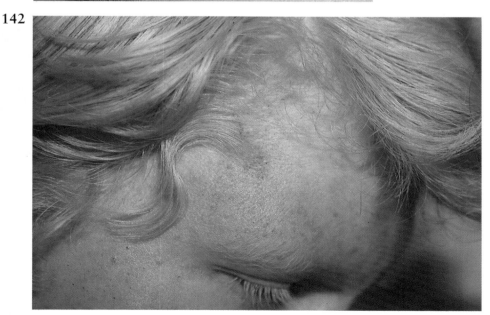

142 Albino. In albinism there is a genetic fault that prevents development of pigment in the hair, skin and eyes. The hair tends to be white or yellowish, the skin burns readily in the sun, and there are often disorders of vision.

Infections and infestations of scalp and hair

Conditions include:

- Ringworm of the scalp.
- Kerion formation.
- Ringworm of the beard and moustache area.
- Favus.
- Pediculosis capitis.

- Phthiriasis pubis.
- Tick bites.
- Trichomycosis axillaris.
- Acne keloid.
- Viral warts.
- Molluscum contagiosum.

Hair and scalp fungal infections

The possibility of fungal infection should always be considered in cases of alopecia with scaling, broken hairs or folliculitis.

In man and some other animals, the fungi that colonize and parasitize keratinized structures are known as dermatophytes. There are three genera: *Microsporum*, *Trichophyton* and *Epidermophyton*. *Epidermophyton* species do not invade hair. Species of *Microsporum* and *Trichophyton* may affect man as their natural host or by accidental transmission: e.g. *Microsporum canis* from cats or dogs and *Trichophyton verrucosum* from cattle. Most types cause only mildly inflamed scaly patches of alopecia with broken off hairs (**143, 145, 148, 149**). The *Trichophyton verrucosum* and *Trichophyton mentagrophytes* species provoke a severe inflammatory reaction in areas with coarse terminal hair. Sometimes it has the appearance of circumscribed folliculitis, but more typically produces kerion morphology (**144, 146, 147**). Kerion starts as a plaque of erythema which becomes oedematous and studded with follicular papules and pustules, and develops as a boggy mass of pustules; it eventually resolves with scarring of the scalp skin and scarring alopecia of variable degree.

The lesions of *Trichophyton schoenleinii* (favus, **148, 149**) vary widely from scaly local patches to large scarred areas, and lesions mimicking psoriasis or seborrhoeic dermatitis.

Diagnosis of fungal infections depends on clinical suspicion, microscopy of plucked hairs and scalp scales, appropriate culture (normally on Sabouraud's medium) and for some species by Wood's light examination in a darkened room. Wood's light (named after the American physicist R.W. Wood) is ultraviolet light passed through glass containing 9% nickel oxide, which is dark purple in colour and screens out visible light. Under Wood's light many species of *Microsporum*, and *Trichophyton schoenleinii*, give off a greenish-blue fluorescence; the former typically show fluorescence of hairs near the scalp, but the latter (favus) shows a duller fluorescence which may be along the whole length of the hairs. Within other *Trichophyton* species fluorescence is variable.

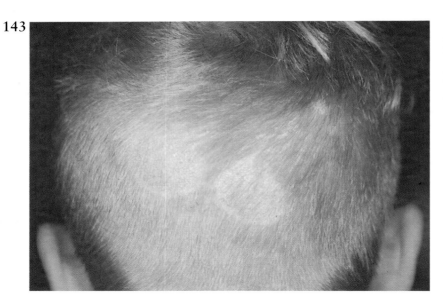

143 Scalp ringworm. Two scaly patches with broken off hair within them are seen, due to *Microsporum canis*, the ringworm that usually affects dogs and cats.

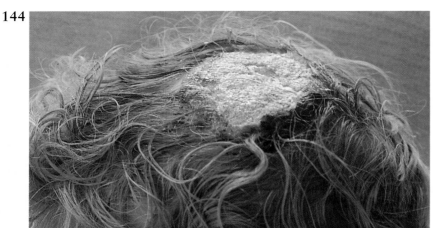

144 Cattle ringworm, scalp kerion type (*Trichophyton verrucosum*).

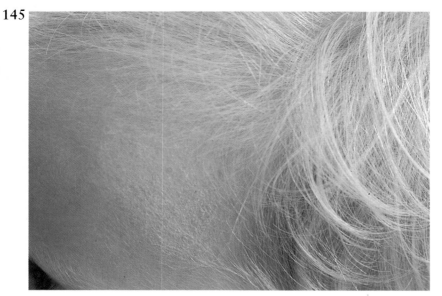

145 Scaly ringworm due to same organism as in **144**, away from hairy area; brother of patient in **144**.

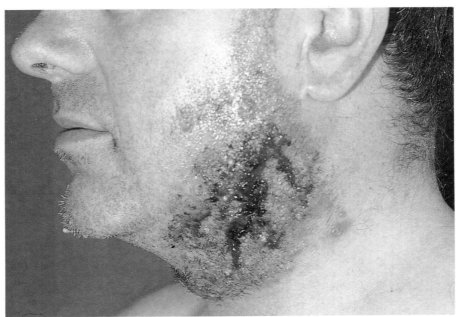

146 Ringworm kerion of the beard area due to infection with the zoophilic fungus *Trichophyton verrucosum* from cattle. This severely inflammatory, sometimes granulomatous or pustular, lesion usually lasts a few months before spontaneous resolution occurs. Similar changes may be produced by *Trichophyton mentagrophytes*, or more rarely by *Trichophyton quinckeanum* from infected mice. (Occasionally *Trichophyton rubrum* infection can produce this type of inflammatory reaction.)

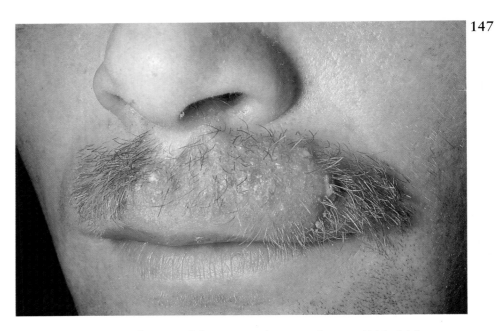

147 Tinea corporis: kerion of the moustache area also see (**144, 146**).

148

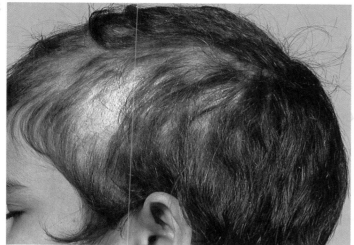

148 Favus, before treatment. Multiple, slightly scaly lesions with broken off hairs are seen, due to the anthrophilic fungus *Trichophyton schoenleinii*. Affected hairs give a dull green fluorescence under Wood's light. Many cases of favus persist for many years and may cause scarring alopecia; lesions on glabrous (non-scalp) skin are more likely to clear spontaneously.

149

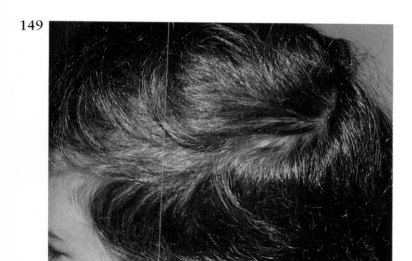

149 Favus: same patient as in **148**, 6 weeks after treatment.

150

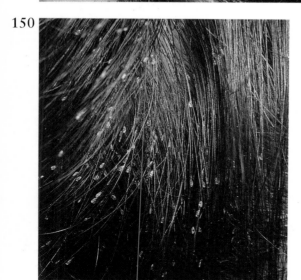

150 Pediculosis capitis (see also **151**). Many ova capsules are seen attached to the affected hairs.

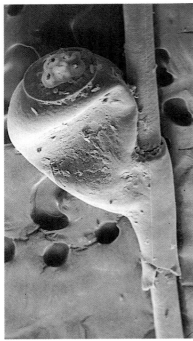

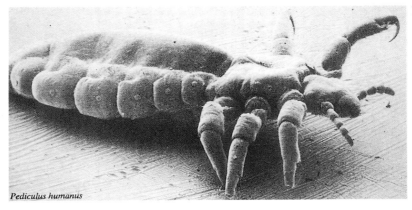

152 *Pediculus humanus* louse. The *Pediculus humanus capitis* form affects the scalp, and *Pediculus humanus corporis* the body. It is probable that the body louse evolved from the head louse, and they may interbreed (scanning EM).

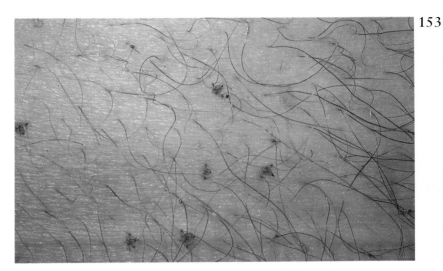

153

151 Pediculosis capitis. An egg capsule (nit) is seen firmly attached to the affected hair shaft. Note the oval capsular lid at the top (scanning EM).

153 *Phthiriasis pubis* (pubic lice, crab lice). Several lice are seen, as well as nits (eggs) stuck to hairs in the lower part of this picture. They usually inhabit the pubic hair, but in hairy individuals will colonize abdominal hair (as seen here), chest hair, beard and moustache, hair, and eyebrows and eyelash hair. Often, close inspection is needed to make the diagnosis.

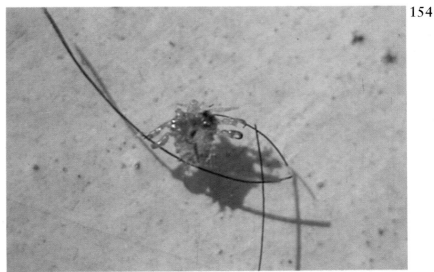

154

154 *Phthirus pubis*. Pubic louse showing method of attachment to hairs.

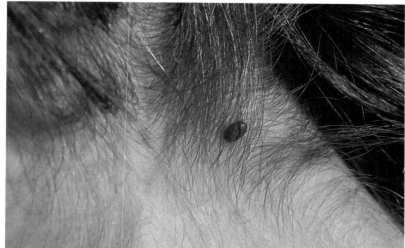

155 **155 Engorged sheep tick, occipital area,** in a child who acquired the tick from an affected dog. A focal (temporary) patch of alopecia may occur, spreading well beyond the inflammation induced, possibly due to anti-coagulants in the tick saliva.

156

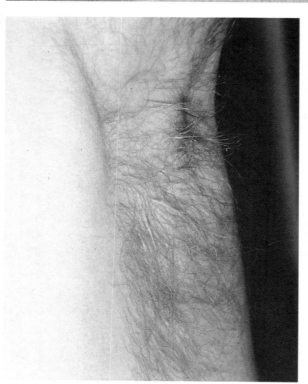

157

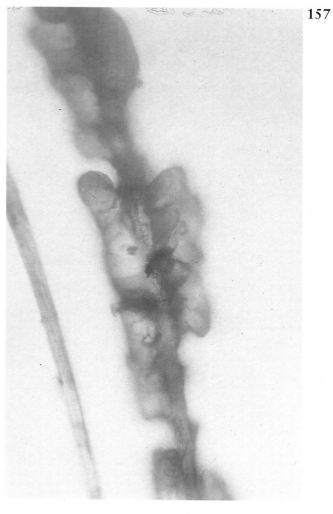

156 Trichomycosis axillaris, sometimes called sticky armpit disease. The concretions attached to axillary hairs are generally accepted as large colonies of the diphtheroid *Corynebacterium tenuis*. It has recently been suggested that the concretions are masses of dried apocrine sweat, since red, yellow and black forms occur and these colours appear in some patients in apocrine sweat without hair infection; i.e. the bacteria are simply colonizing these deposits. The affected hairs fluoresce a pale red-pink colour.

157 Trichomycosis axillaris (light micrograph): concretions around a single hair.

158 Trichomycosis axillaris: transmission EM, showing large numbers of bacteria surrounding loose cuticular cells. Note the absence of invasion of the cortex on the right.

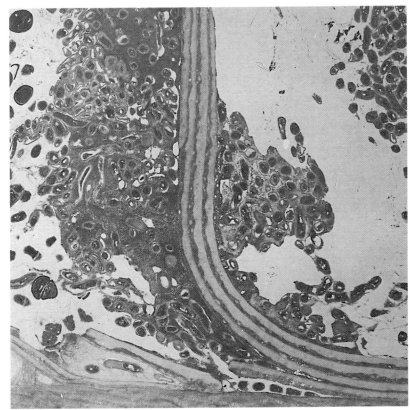

159 Acne keloid (nuchae). Progressive occipital scarring in a nodular or plaque form occurs following episodes of follicular pustulation, a distinctive scarring process peculiar to negroid male individuals.

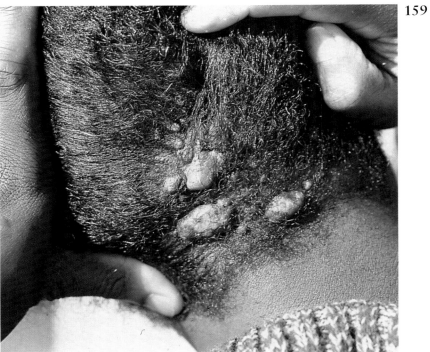

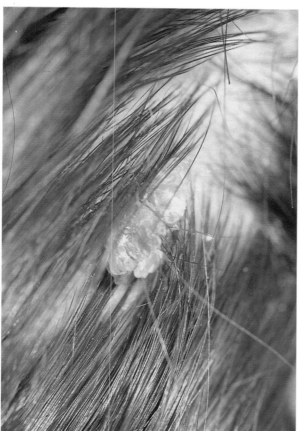

160 Viral wart. Viral warts of the scalp tend to be papillomatous and keratotic.

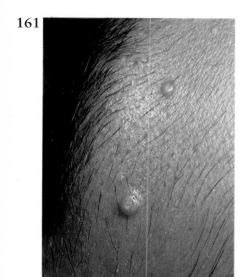

161 Molluscum contagiosum. Characteristic umbilicated papules are seen.

Hair and scalp in systemic diseases

Infections include:

- Lepromatous leprosy.
- Secondary syphilis.
- *Nocardia*.
- *Varicella/zoster*.

Other diseases include:

- Post-febrile diffuse alopecia.
- Iron deficiency diffuse alopecia.
- Zinc deficiency (acrodermatitis entero-pathica type).
- Systemic lupus erythematosus.
- Dermatomyositis.
- Giant cell arteritis.
- Langerhans' cell histiocytosis.

162 Lepromatous leprosy. Loss of hairs from the eyebrows is seen, a common feature. Whether diffuse scalp alopecia, which sometimes accompanies leprosy, is a specific feature of it or a non-specific telogen effluvium is not known.

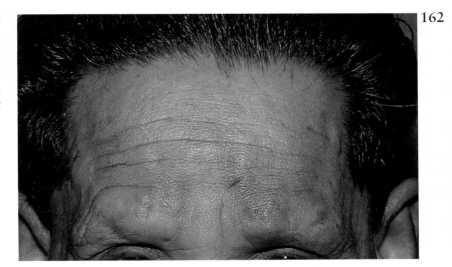

162

163 Secondary syphilis, showing diffuse scalp hair loss mimicking alopecia areata. The alopecia may appear patchy, giving a moth-eaten appearance, particularly in the occipital area.

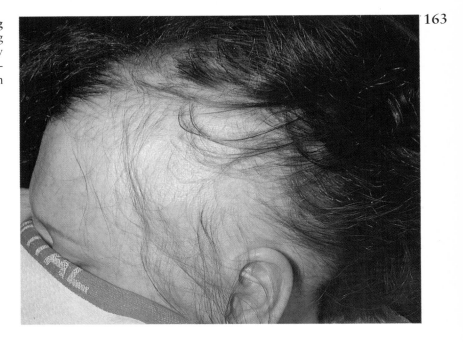

163

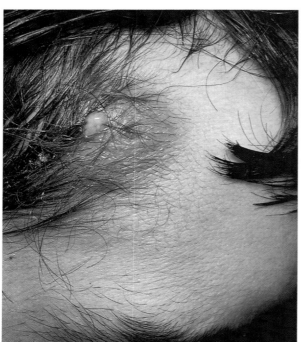

164 *Nocardia* infection of the scalp in a patient being treated for Hodgkin's disease. Such lesions may occur in any patient with severe immunosuppression from disease or drugs.

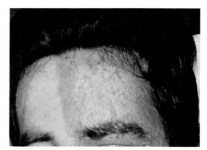

165 *Herpes zoster,* affecting the ophthalmic division of the trigeminal nerve. Lesions extend into the scalp.

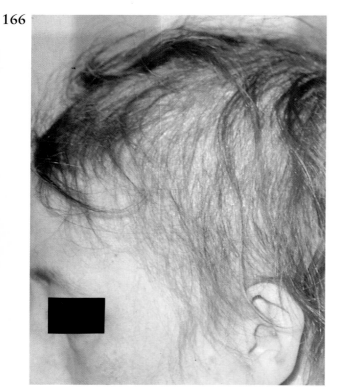

166 Post-febrile diffuse alopecia, telogen effluvium **type,** due to severe respiratory infection.

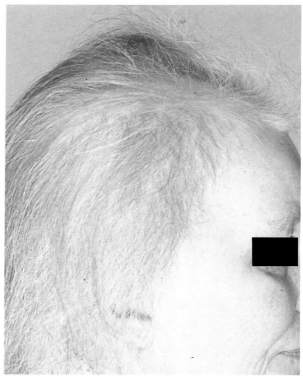

167 Diffuse alopecia, telogen effluvium **type,** in this patient due to chronic iron deficiency resulting from peptic ulcer and aspirin administration.

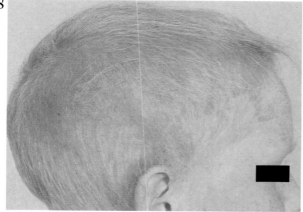 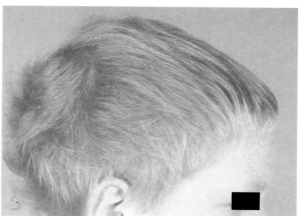

168, 169 Zinc deficiency of acrodermatitis enteropathica type. Diffuse alopecia is seen before (**168**) and improving after (**169**) zinc therapy. This patient, only diagnosed at 10 years of age, also had photophobia, a peripheral psoriasiform rash, and multiple Beau's lines on finger and toe nails.

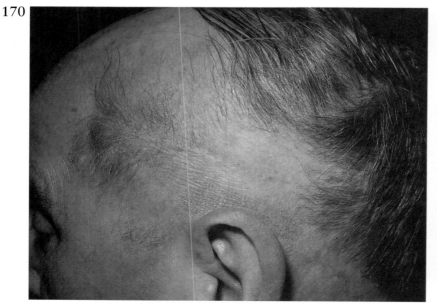 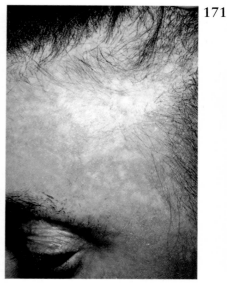

170 Systemic lupus erythematosus. There is considerable hair loss on a background of erythema, telangiectasia and scarring.

171 Dermatomyositis, scarring alopecia. Chronic dermatomyositis in young people can produce considerable scarring.

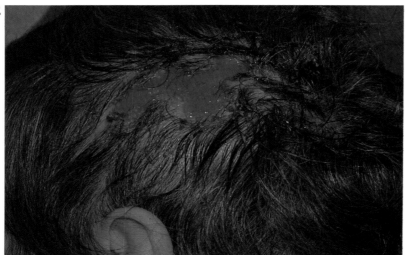

172 Giant cell arteritis: a unilateral parietal prominent erosion is seen in the distribution of the temporal artery. Pain is variable, but associated features are unilateral sudden blindness, fever and malaise. The temporal arteries are always easily palpable. Sometimes muscle and joint pains are associated. The erythrocyte sedimentation rate is always raised, often above 100 mm in one hour. Temporal artery biopsy is required, and is usually diagnostic.

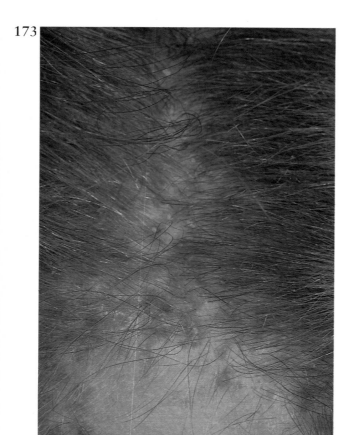

173 Langerhan's cell histiocytosis (histiocytosis X), affecting the scalp; there is an eruption of granular scaly indurated papules with slight surface scaling. At first sight it may resemble seborrhoeic dermatitis or bacterial folliculitis. This type may occur in isolation or in association with other classical skin and systemic changes; e.g. diabetes insipidus, proptosis, spontaneous pneumothoraces, xanthelasmata, and bony lesions due to eosinophilic granuloma. This condition has been variously called Hand–Schüller–Christian disease, Letterer–Siwe disease, and eosinophilic granuloma, but they are all manifestations of proliferation of Langerhan's cells. (Courtesy Dr. A. du Vivier.)

Skin diseases affecting the scalp and hair

Conditions include:

- Pityriasus capitis (dandruff).
- Pityriasis amiantacea.
- Seborrhoeic dermatitis.
- Atopic dermatitis.
- Allergic contact dermatitis.
- Lichen simplex.
- Psoriasis.
- Pityriasis rubra pilaris.

- Folliculitis cheloidalis nuchae.
- Pseudofolliculitis.
- Follicular mucinosis.
- Discoid lupus erythematosus.
- Darier's disease.
- Pemphigus vulgaris.
- Cicatricial pemphigoid.
- Fox–Fordyce disease.
- Hidradenitis suppurativa.
- Elastoma perforans serpiginosa.

174 Pityriasis capitis (dandruff). There is diffuse fine scaling without any inflammation. Sometimes the scalp is itchy. This is best regarded as the pre-inflammatory stage of seborrhoeic dermatitis. Scalp yeasts (*Pityrosporum ovale*) are invariably found in large numbers.

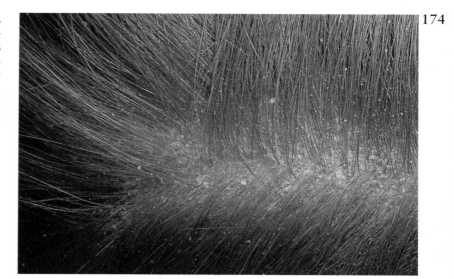

174

175 Pityriasis capitis in a patient with seborrhoeic dermatitis, with many peripilar keratin casts surrounding hairs; these excrescences have been called pseudo-nits.

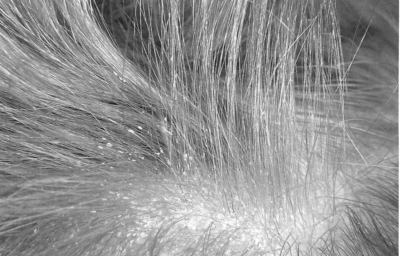

175

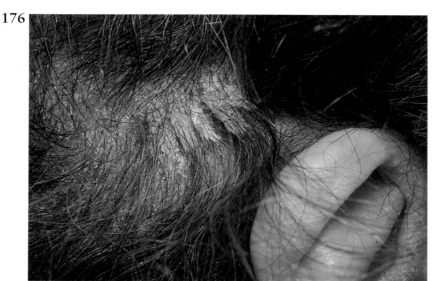

176 **Pityriasis amiantacea** here showing adherent scale surrounding and attached to the proximal part of groups of hairs. This condition may occur in isolation, generally being considered within the seborrheoic spectrum of diseases; however, similar changes may occur in psoriasis and even, occasionally, in lichen planus of the scalp.

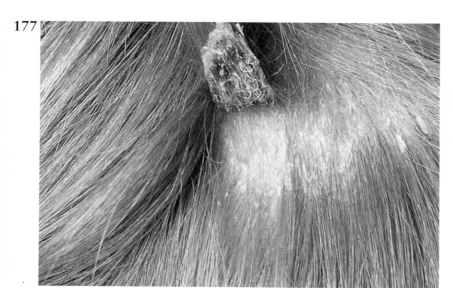

177 **Pityriasis ('tinea') amiantacea** (see also **176**). Thick adherent scales develop, particularly on the vertex around the base of the hairs and sleeving them with keratin. Sometimes, as here, whole locks of hair are enmeshed with underlying hair loss, which is usually temporary.

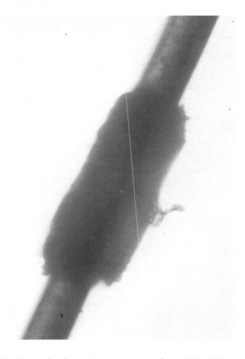

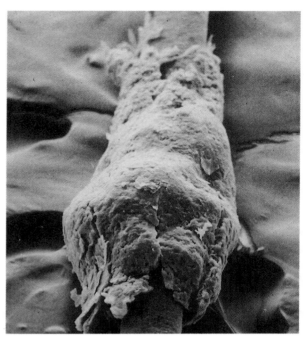

178 Peripilar keratin casts (see also **175,179**): light micrograph. The cast is surrounding, but not attached to, the hair shaft.

179 Peripilar keratin cast (scanning EM), clearly showing that the cast is not attached to the underlying normal hair. This keratinous cast is formed within the hair follicle infundibulum, either from the epidermis at that site or from the internal root sheath, which fails to desquamate in the usual way from the follicular opening.

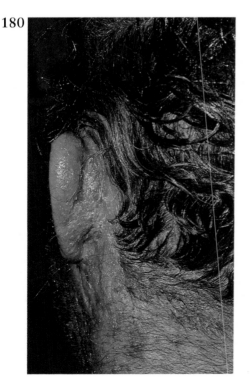

180 Seborrhoeic dermatitis of the scalp, neck and ear. This condition is associated with the presence of *Pityrosporum* yeasts, but the scaling and crusting seen here suggest secondary bacterial infection.

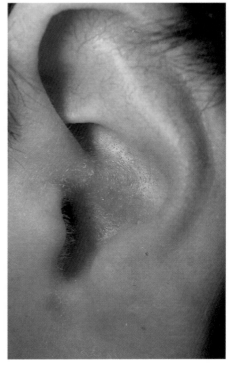

181 Seborrhoeic dermatitis of the ears, showing redness and scaling within the helix. This is one form of otitis externa, which can also result from atopic dermatitis, allergic contact dermatitis, and from chronic middle ear discharge.

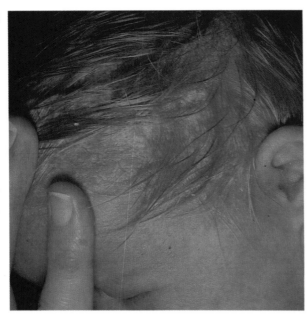

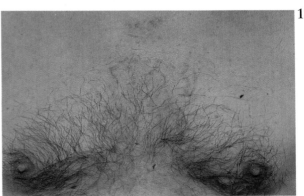

183 Seborrhoeic dermatitis of the presternal hairy skin.

182 Seborrhoeic dermatitis of infancy affecting the scalp, ear and face. Distinction from atopic dermatitis at this age may be difficult.

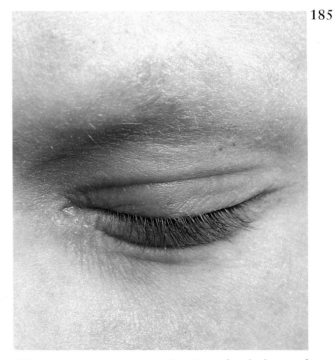

184 Atopic dermatitis. Intensely pruritic face and scalp atopic dermatitis is common at all ages, but particularly pronounced in infants and children.

185 Atopic dermatitis, showing focal loss of eyebrow hair probably due to weathering from rubbing and/or scratching. Lichenification of the eyelids is also well shown.

186 Atopic dermatitis: acute dermatitis of the fronto-temporal area and the ear. The scalp, face and neck are common sites of involvement in this condition.

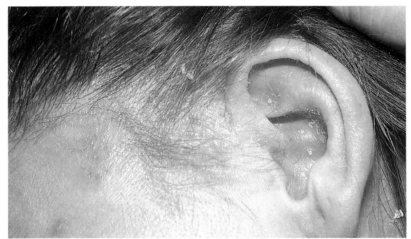

187 Atopic dermatitis: severe involvement of the neck and adjacent scalp with lichenification, erosions and hair loss.

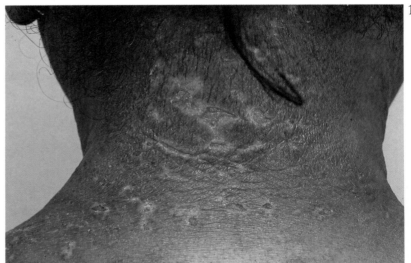

188 Allergic contact dermatitis, due to paraphenylenediamine hair dye. This clinical picture can be mistaken for angio-oedema. Allergy to products applied to the scalp or hair most typically affects the skin of the hair margins, the eyelids or the face, with the scalp itself being only minimally affected or not at all.

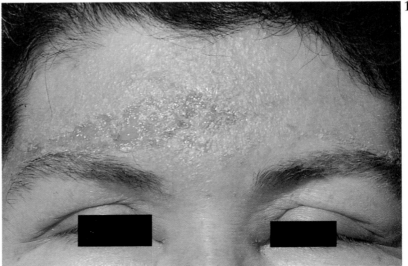

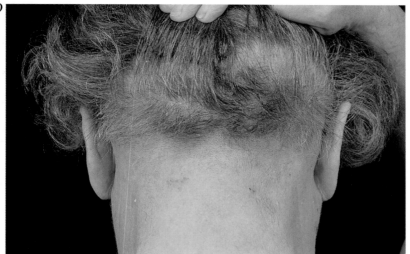

189 Allergic contact dermatitis in the nuchal area, in this case due to nail varnish allergy.

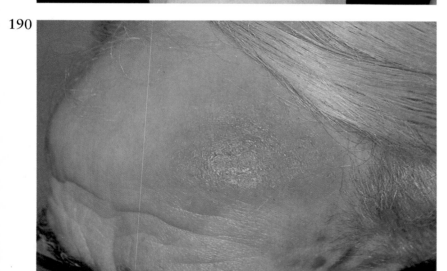

190 Forehead: allergic contact dermatitis. This eruption was due to a chemical in a hat band. Possible allergens include dyes and chromate.

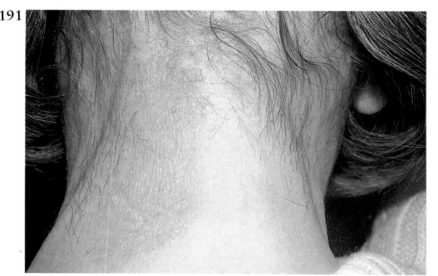

191 Lichen simplex of the posterior hair margin: lichenification due to constant rubbing and scratching in a classical site. This nuchal type is more common in women.

192 Psoriasis of the scalp. Red scaly lesions can be seen at the scalp margin and within the scalp; there is a sharp margin between affected and unaffected skin.

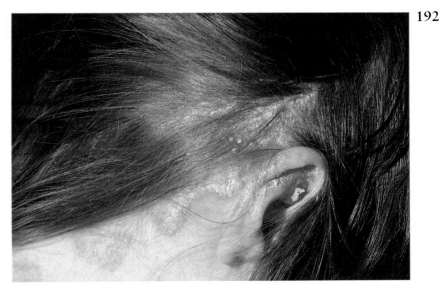

193 Psoriasis of the scalp, frontal scaling visible in this case at the hair margin.

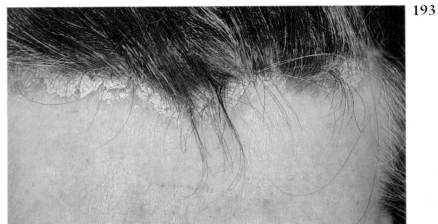

194 Psoriasis of the scalp: a patch affecting the nape of the neck with severe scaling and many peripilar keratin casts.

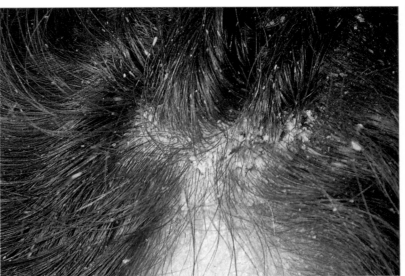

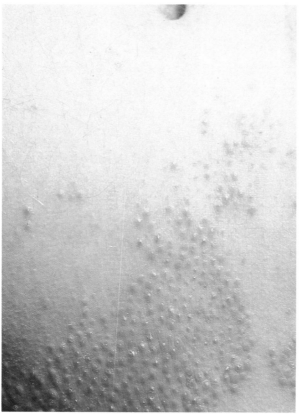

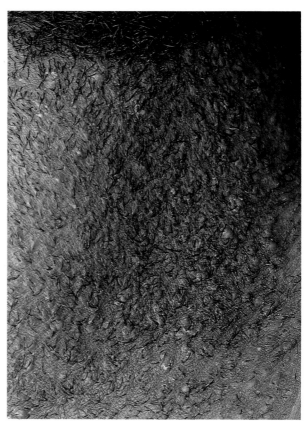

195 Pityriasis rubra pilaris. This persistent wide-spread scaly eruption of unknown cause is characterized by individual red, follicular, keratotic lesions often, as here, within sharply marginated plaques. The follicular pattern is not always so prominent, and the appearance is then more like that of seborrhoeic dermatitis or psoriasis.

196 Pseudofolliculitis barbae of the beard area. Most often seen in negroid subjects with tightly curling hair, this papular inflammatory condition relates to hair shafts coiling and curving back into the skin and provoking an inflammatory reaction. Secondary bacterial infection may be present.

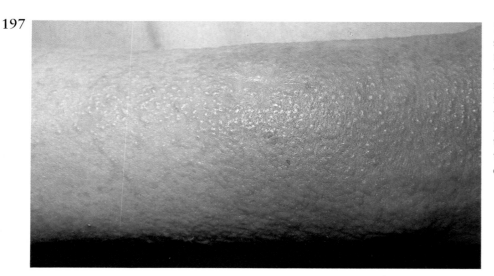

197 Follicular mucinosis: an infiltrated erythematous plaque of the arm with prominent follicular involvement and hair loss, in this case associated with mycosis fungoides. Many cases, particularly those in childhood and with isolated lesions, are entirely benign.

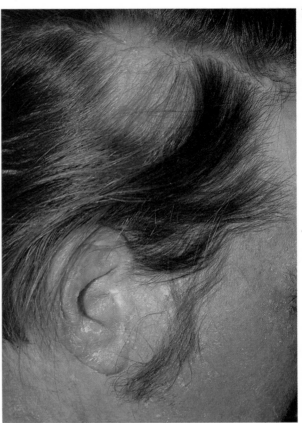

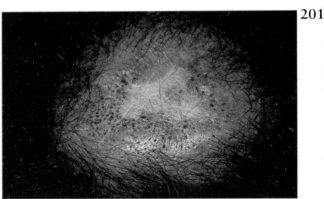

198 Discoid lupus erythematosus. Typical centrally scarred lesions with marginal active inflammation, affecting the face and scalp.

199 Discoid lupus erythematosus: a less actively inflamed lesion with scarring alopecia.

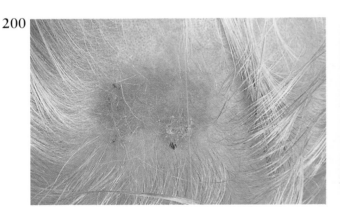

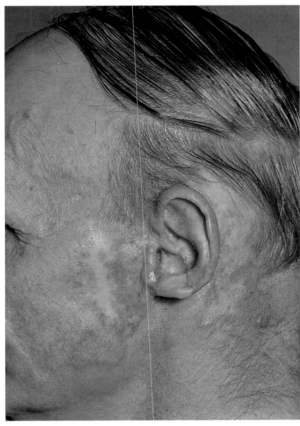

200 Discoid lupus erythematosus: a single lesion of the scalp; an earlier and more inflammatory phase than in 198.

201 Discoid lupus erythematosus in a negroid subject: a single lesion showing central scarring and pigment loss and a peripheral hyperpigmented inflammatory area containing prominent follicular plugging (hyperkeratosis).

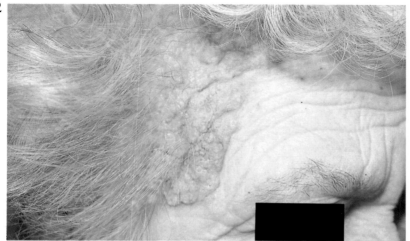

202 Darier's disease: extensive scalp involvement with, in this case, considerable dyskeratotic thickening. Hair loss is less common with scalp lesions than at other sites (e.g. **204**).

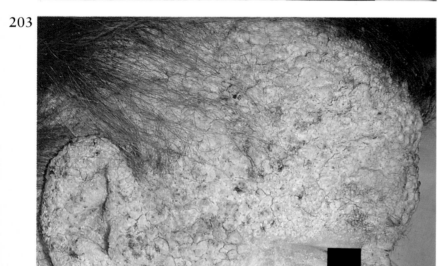

203 Darier's disease: severe form, affecting face and scalp.

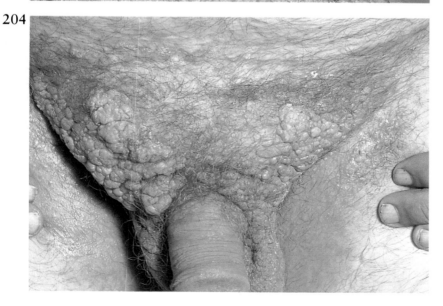

204 Darier's disease, pubic hair area. Warty, often secondarily infected lesions (bacterial or viral) in the crural area with marked hair loss. This dominantly inherited defect of keratinization (synonym, keratosis follicularis) may not be fully manifest until adult life, although minor signs can occur in childhood.

205 Pemphigus vulgaris of the scalp, showing erosions, crusting and hair loss in the affected areas.

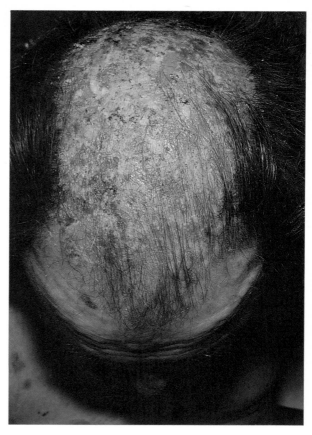

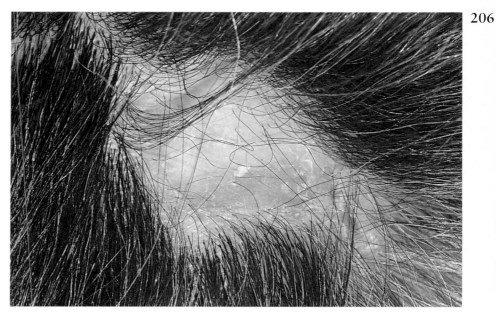

206 Cicatricial pemphigoid: areas of inflammatory scarring alopecia of the scalp are associated with blisters and scarring of the mouth, conjunctival sac, and other skin sites, particularly the ano-genital area. Sometimes webs of scarring occur in the pharynx and oesophagus.

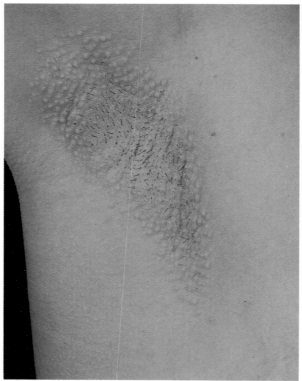

207 Fox–Fordyce disease, showing dome-shaped axillary papules. This apocrine inflammatory eruption may cause considerable pruritus and is the apocrine duct equivalent of eccrine gland prickly heat. It is commonest in young adult women.

208 Hidradenitis suppurativa, axilla: severe androgen-dependent apocrine infection and inflammation with hair loss.

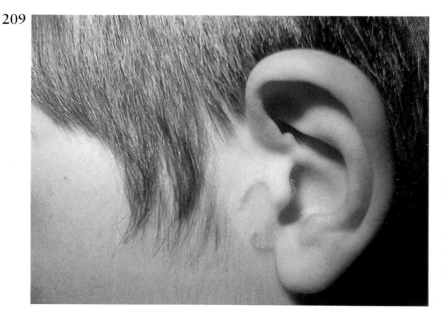

209 Elastoma perforans serpiginosa. This rare condition may occur in normal individuals, but is usually seen in those with inherited or acquired connective tissue abnormalities, e.g. in Down's syndrome or in patients receiving penicillamine therapy. The individual lesions, mostly on the head and neck, start as papules (sometimes warty), which extend to become grouped in circles or arcs. The diagnosis is confirmed by the histological appearance, which shows focal increase of large elastic fibres which in the necrotic lesion are seen to be extruded through the overlying epidermis (transepithelial extrusion of dermal tissue).

Naevi, cysts and tumours of the scalp

Conditions include:

- Naevus flammeus.
- Strawberry naevus.
- Naevus sebaceous.
- Nodular sebaceous naevus.
- Pilomatrixoma.
- Cylindroma (turban tumour).
- Syringocystadenoma papilliferum.
- Basal cell naevus syndrome (Gorlin's syndrome).
- Becker's naevus.
- Hair follicle naevus.
- Compound melanocytic naevus.
- Cellular blue naevus.
- Epidermoid cyst.
- Pilar (trichilemmal) cyst.
- Post-auricular pilar cyst.

- Inclusion dermoid cyst.
- Xanthoma.
- Fibroepithelial polyp.
- Campbell de Morgan spot (cherry angioma).
- Pyogenic granuloma.
- Seborrhoeic keratosis.
- Trichofolliculoma.
- Actinic keratosis.
- Cutaneous horn.
- Keratoacanthoma.
- Squamous carcinoma.
- Alopecia neoplastica.
- Basal cell carcinoma.
- Metastasis.
- Lentigo maligna melanoma.
- Mycosis fungoides.
- B-cell lymphoma.

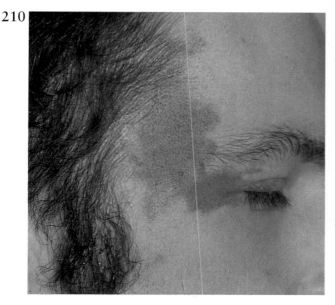

210 Naevus flammeus (port wine stain). This flat, segmental, unilateral vascular naevus is common on the upper face and scalp, as in this example. The rare association of this naevus with ocular and intracranial angiomatosis is known as the Sturge–Weber syndrome (it results in ocular defects, grand mal epilepsy and often contralateral limb paralysis). This naevus shows no propensity for spontaneous resolution; compare strawberry vascular angiomata.

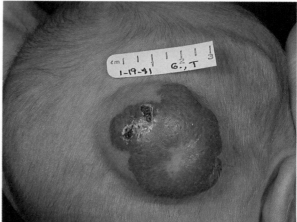

211 Strawberry naevus (cavernous haemangioma) of scalp. Such lesions are more common in girls, beginning during the first months of life and continuing to enlarge, often up to 2 to 3 years of age. Most lesions involute spontaneously by 5 years of age, leaving little or no scarring. During infancy superficial ulceration may occur, occasionally associated with bacterial infection.

212

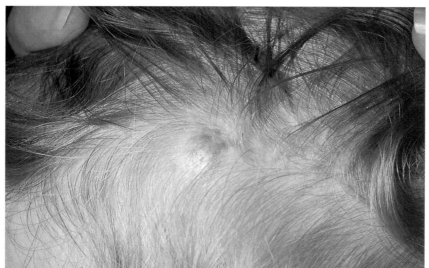

212 Strawberry naevus of the scalp, a resolving lesion (compare earlier figures).

213

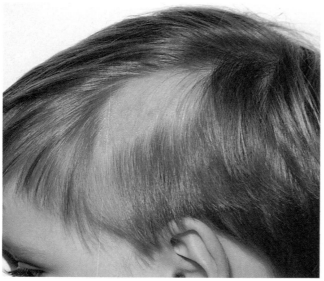

213 Naevus sebaceous involving the scalp. The majority of these naevi are on the scalp or face. Typically yellowish-brown in colour, the lesion is usually slightly elevated and velvety to the touch.

214

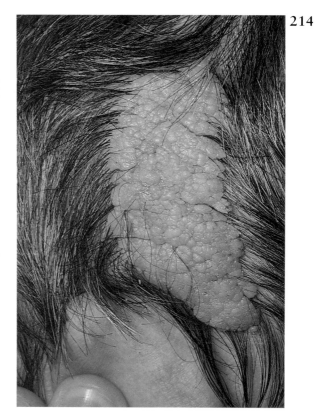

214 Naevus sebaceous of the scalp, adjacent to the ear. Thickened and raised lesions such as this are more prominent after puberty, owing to androgenic stimulation of the sebaceous gland component. Basal cell carcinoma may develop in these lesions during adult life.

215 Basal cell carcinoma in naevus sebaceous.

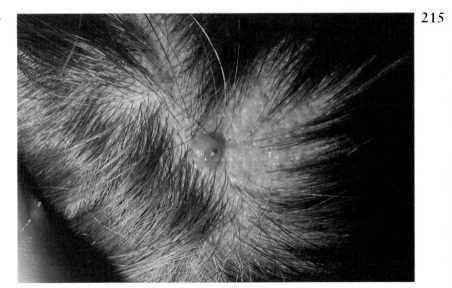

216 Nodular sebaceous naevus, nodular sebaceous adenomatous type.

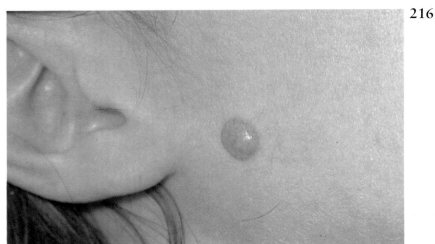

217 Sebaceous gland hypertrophy (forehead). These small, harmless crateriform lesions occur from middle age onwards. They are skin coloured or yellowish, but if blood vessels are prominent in the margin they can be mistaken for basal cell carcinomas.

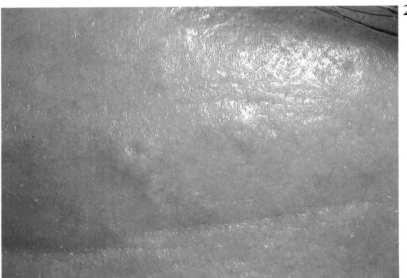

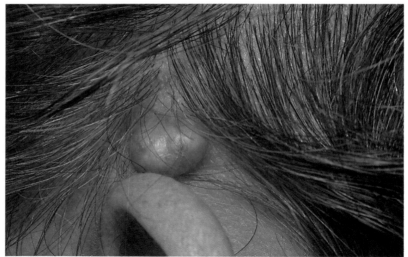

218 Pilomatrixoma, a nodular tumour of the matrix cells of the hair bulb, here seen on the scalp. Such tumours are usually solitary; in published series of cases 6% to 12% were on the scalp.

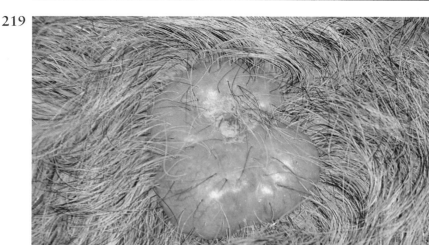

219 Cylindroma (dermal cylindroma, turban tumour, Spiegler's tumour). This tumour is rare, but often familial, and tends to affect young women. The scalp is the most frequent site. Occasionally multiple lesions and large hairless lobular masses develop. They have a characteristic histology.

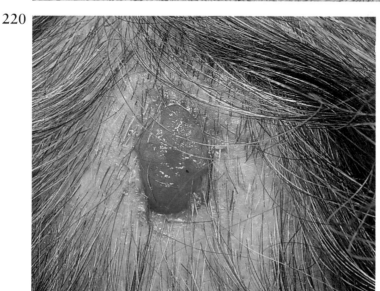

220 Syringocystadenoma papilliferum. This naevoid condition may occur as part of a more complex naevus or show more or less specific apocrine sweat gland differentiation. This typical scalp lesion is red and nodular; about 50% occur in the scalp, developing in infancy or early childhood.

221 Basal cell naevus syndrome (Gorlin's syndrome): multiple polymorphic naevoid basal cell carcinomas on the scalp and ear. These tumours may show atypical morphology; therefore, any new nodule or indurated lesion should be considered tumorous. Whatever surgical method is adopted for removal, histological examination is needed.

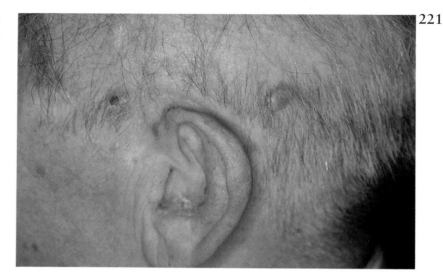

222 Becker's naevus (acquired hairy pigmental epidermal naevus). This unilateral segmental naevus is commonly found on the upper trunk; increasing pigmentation starts in late childhood and rather coarse hairs develop after puberty. It is possible that the affected area of skin has enhanced androgen receptor activity, which explains the onset at puberty and the presence of acne vulgaris in the lesion.

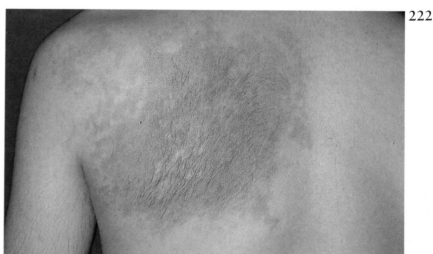

223 Hair follicle naevus (*not* a Becker's naevus). Localized hypertrichosis, resulting from a naevus of large follicles with no other abnormality, is not uncommon.

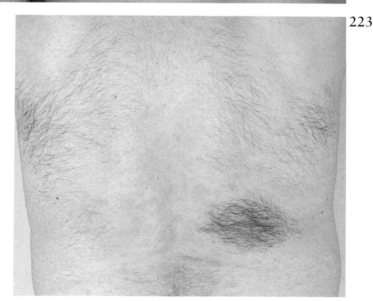

224

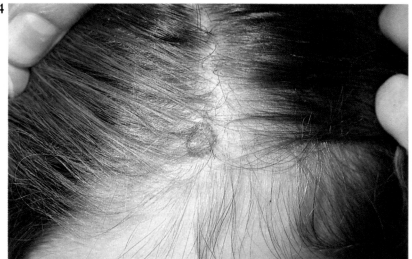

224 Compound melanocytic naevus. Such soft nodules, variably pigmented, are common on the scalp; patients often ask for them to be removed because of their susceptibility to minor trauma. Coarser hair than in surrounding skin may be associated.

225

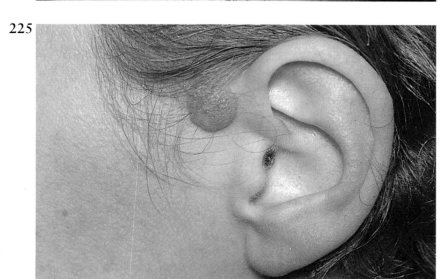

225 Benign compound melanocytic naevus. These lesions are soft, give rise to no symptoms (unless traumatized) and have no malignant potential. Pigmentation is variable from lesion to lesion.

226

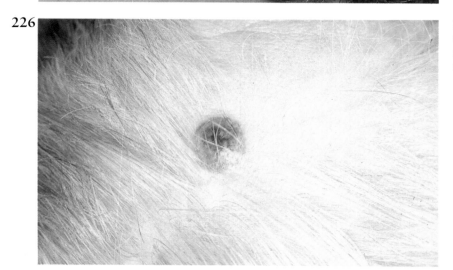

226 Cellular blue naevus of the scalp: a common site for this deep melanocytic naevus. Malignant transformation rarely occurs.

227 Epidermoid cysts of the scalp, here associated with overlying hair loss. These lesions are often miscalled sebaceous cysts.

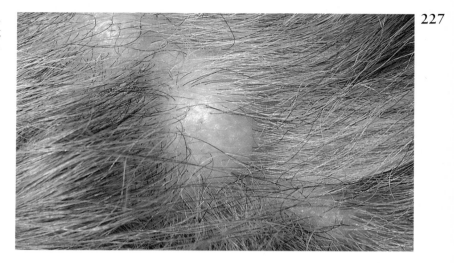

227

228 Pilar (trichilemmal) cyst of the scalp. Derived from the hair root sheath, these cysts (also often miscalled sebaceous cysts) are common on the scalp, and vary in size from that of a pea to that of a walnut. They are familial, and are more common in women.

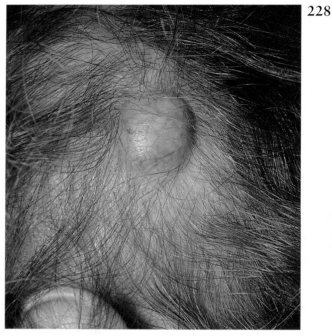

228

229 Post-auricular pilar cysts: a relatively common finding in hidradenitis suppurativa and acne conglobata.

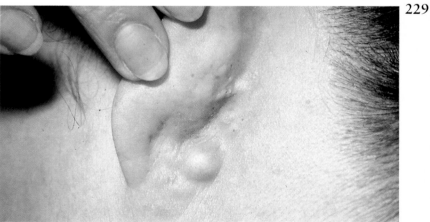

229

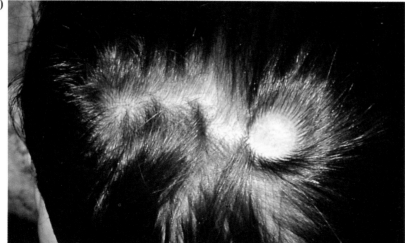

230 Congenital inclusion dermoid cyst with absent hair occurring occipitally at a suture line of the cranial bones. The cyst may not be obvious clinically, and may present as focal absence of hair. However, the changes are clearly evident on histology.

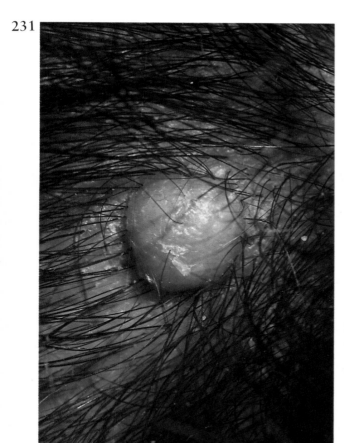

231 Xanthoma. This is a solitary lesion in an otherwise healthy individual. Hyperlipidaemia should be excluded.

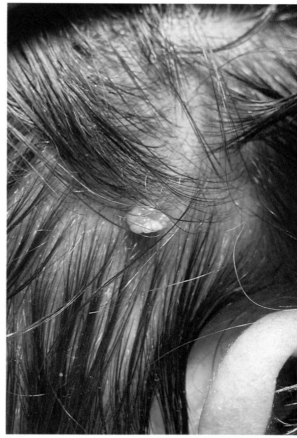

232 Papillomatous benign fibroepithelial polyp in the scalp. These are not uncommon in the scalp, and are frequently subject to minor trauma.

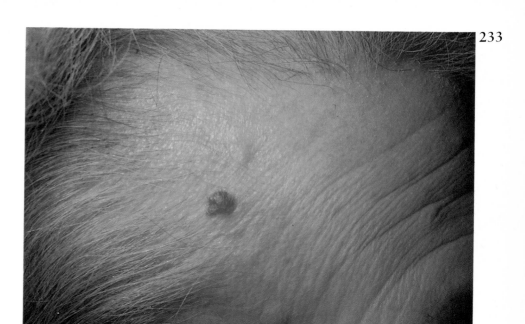

233 Campbell de Morgan spot (cherry angioma). These tiny red angiomas are common on the trunk after middle life, and occur not infrequently on the scalp.

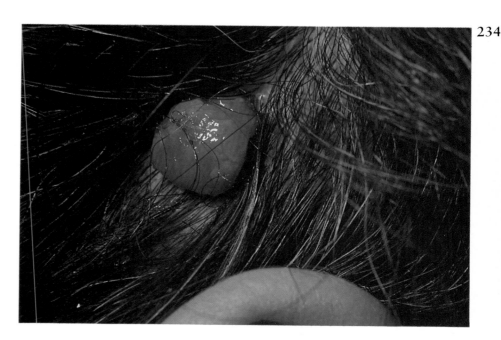

234 Pyogenic granuloma of the scalp. These lesions are bright red, soft vascular nodules of variable size, and either ulcerated or with intact epithelium. Bleeding on minor trauma is very common. Lesions can last for months or years if untreated. The nodule consists of hyperplastic vascular tissue (surgical granulation tissue). Often following minor trauma, it is not primarily due to infection. Scalp metastases can have an identical appearance, and histology is always required.

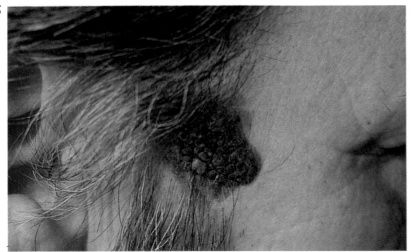

235 Seborrhoeic keratosis. These are common warty lesions of middle and old age (synonyms: basal cell papilloma; seborrhoeic wart). Microscopically the epidermis is thickened with a solid epithelial mass, resembling basal cells, forming flat, serrated or retiform patterns with horn cysts or pseudocysts. The lesions may occur anywhere on the body where pilosebaceous units exist, but most commonly on the face, scalp and trunk. They start as small flat papules, skin coloured or slightly brown. They may increase in numbers and remain small or become large (up to several centimetres diameter), with increasing darkening until they are jet black. The surface is usually soft and finely lobulated, and often appears greasy. If large numbers occur pruritus may be a problem. They have no capacity to become malignant.

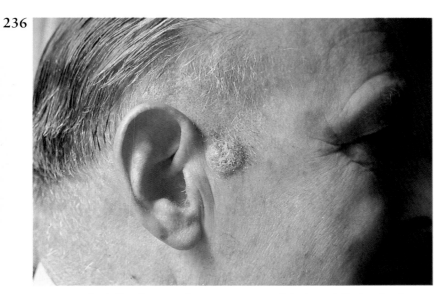

236 Trichofolliculoma. A benign tumour of the hair follicle which may mimic molluscum contagiosum, keratoacanthoma, squamous epithelioma, or actinic keratoses. It presents as a solitary dome-shaped nodule with a central pore through which a wool-like tuft of hair projects.

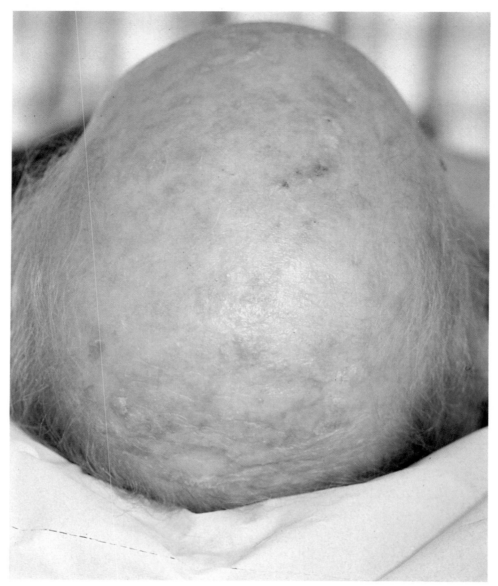

237 Diffuse solar atrophy and actinic keratoses. Solar (actinic) keratoses are common lesions of all exposed skin, including the bald or balding scalp. The more fair-skinned the individual and the greater the amount of sun exposure, the more likely are these lesions to occur. Initially lesions may be patches of roughness, often red or pigmented. Later, well demarcated horny crusts of varying size develop, sometimes with associated inflammation and pigmentation. The balding scalp or chronically sun damaged face may develop them in larger numbers. Transformation to squamous carcinoma can occur, at which stage irregular underlying or surrounding induration develops. Histologically the surface hyperkeratosis is always associated with some degree of dermal solar elastosis; the differentiating epidermis becomes disorderly and may be either thinned or acanthotic.

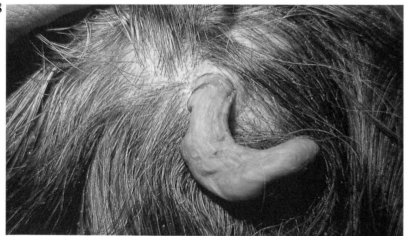

238 Cutaneous horn of the scalp. This is an unusually large example. Such lesions are usually benign, but the base of the lesion may show epidermal cell dysplasia or early, well differentiated, squamous carcinoma change.

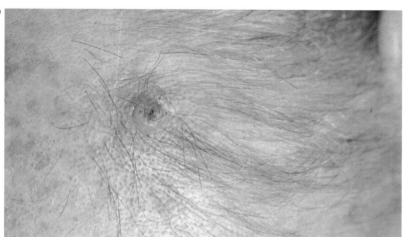

239 Keratoacanthoma: a small lesion on the scalp.

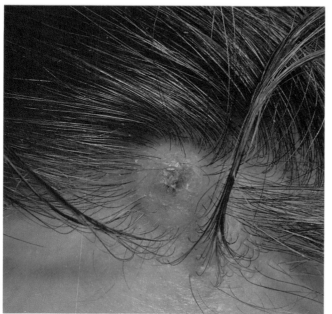

240 Keratoacanthoma, at frontal hair margin.

241 Keratoacanthoma, histology (239, 240). This self-limiting lesion is a relatively common tumour of the skin occurring in the same susceptible populations in whom squamous epithelioma is found, but in a younger age group. It is thought to be of follicular (infundibular) origin. Histologically the overall architecture is usually diagnostic; a central horny mass is surrounded by columns of orderly hyperplastic epithelium with many mitoses visible. There is a mixed monocytic infiltrate underlying the tumour. Clinically the evolution is often alarming; a hemispherical papule occurs, enlarging rapidly to reach up to 1 to 2 cms or more within 4 to 6 weeks; further enlargement is rare. After a further 6 to 8 weeks the lesion regresses, sheds its central horny core, and finally resolves spontaneously, leaving only a puckered scar. If the diagnosis is in doubt, it should be removed as a suspected squamous carcinoma.

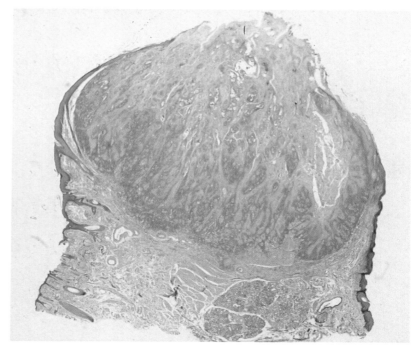

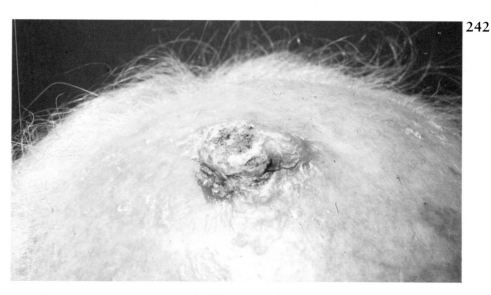

242 Squamous carcinoma: a well differentiated type on the bald scalp with an irregular keratotic surface.

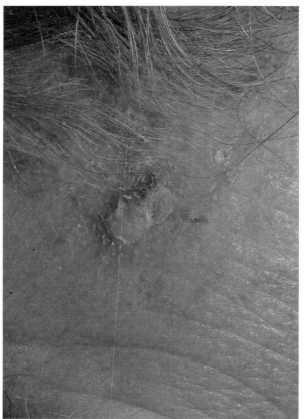

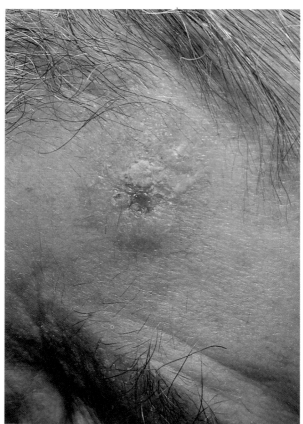

243 Squamous carcinoma. A small, well differentiated type at the hair margin. Since such lesions are mostly associated with ultraviolet radiation damage, they are usually seen in light-exposed areas at the fronto-temporal scalp margins or on the bald scalp.

244 Squamous carcinoma. A well differentiated lesion at the frontal scalp margin. More tumour infiltration is seen than in **243**.

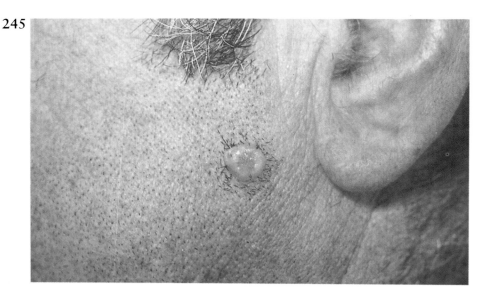

245 Cutaneous squamous cell carcinoma in an immunosuppressed patient following kidney transplant and cyclosporin-A therapy. Sometimes these lesions look like early keratoacanthomas, but they do not remit and may metastasize.

246 Alopecia neoplastica, a type of scarring alopecia due to metastases, e.g. from carcinoma of the breast.

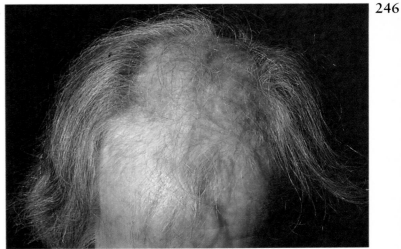

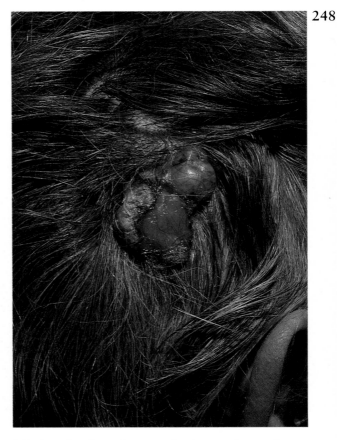

247 Alopecia neoplastica, skin biopsy from patient in 246; lines of metastatic carcinoma cells (arrow) are seen in a dense collagenous stroma.

248 Basal cell carcinoma. This lesion shows ulceration, hyperkeratosis, cyst formation and pigmentation. An important differential diagnosis is malignant melanoma.

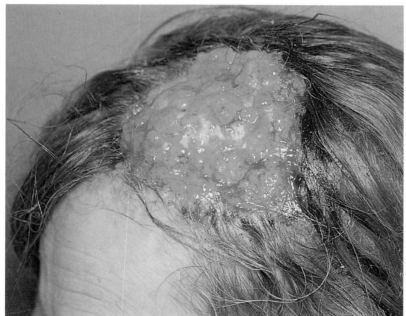

249 Basal cell carcinoma of the scalp: an unusually large, neglected, eroded rodent ulcer type.

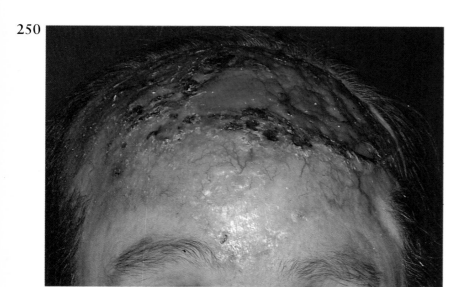

250 Basal cell carcinoma. This very extensive lesion eventually caused death by infiltration through the bones of the skull and invasion of dura and meningeal blood vessels.

251 Basal cell carcinoma. This lesion is large and has pigmented areas.

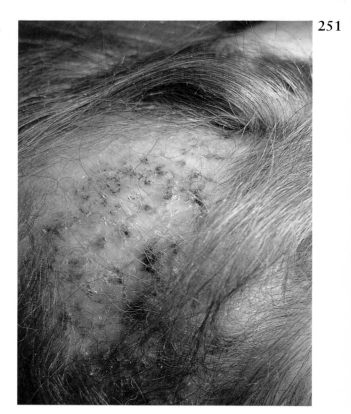

252 Metastasis, scalp, from carcinoma of kidney. This very vascular lesion closely resembles a pyogenic granuloma, but sometimes metastases look more like rather vascular scalp cysts. Undiagnosed scalp lesions require biopsy.

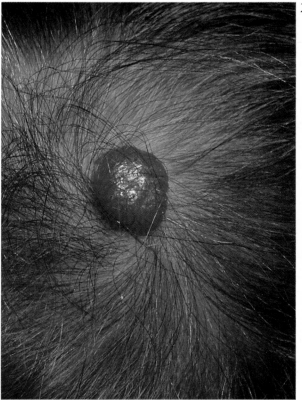

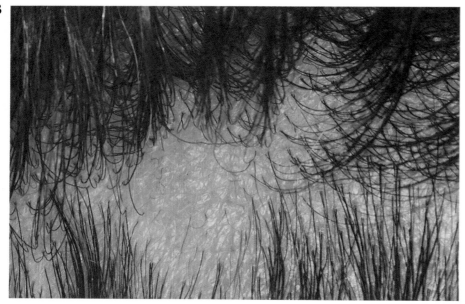

253 Metastasis, scalp, from carcinoma of the breast. This lesion resembled lupus erythematous. Its true nature was revealed by biopsy.

254

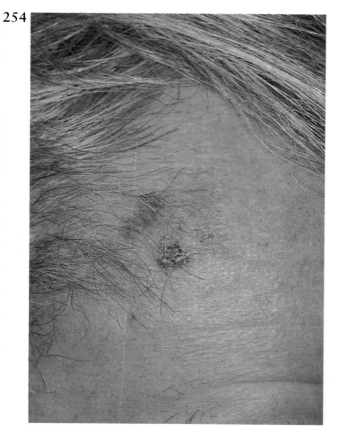

254 Lentigo maligna melanoma: anterior scalp margin.

255 Lentigo maligna in X-ray damaged skin. Radiotherapy had been given for tinea capitis in childhood.

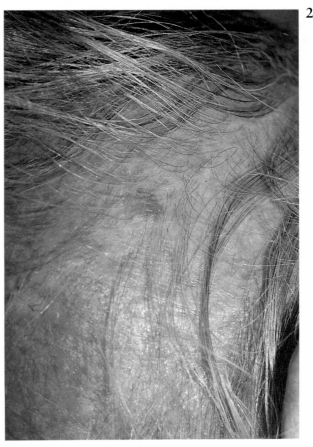

256 Mycosis fungoides, chronic T-cell lymphoma of the skin, here presenting as a tumour with associated hair loss. This type of lesion may show follicular mucinosis histologically.

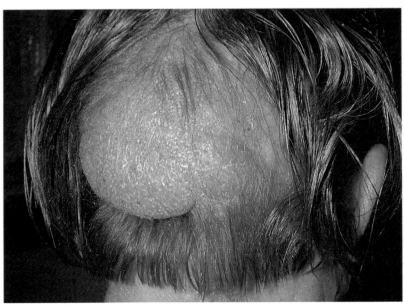

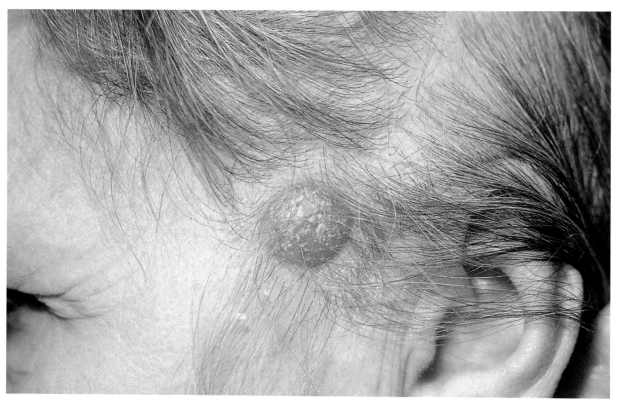

257 B-cell lymphomatous nodule at the scalp margin. Such lesions typically arise on previously normal skin (whereas, in mycosis fungoides, tumours arise in pre-existing scaly plaques).

Nails: anatomy of the nail apparatus

The nail apparatus produces a strong, relatively inflexible, keratinous nail plate over the dorsal surface of the end of each digit which protects the finger tip. By exerting counter-pressure over the volar skin and pulp, the flat nail plate adds to the precision and delicacy of touch, the ability to pick up small objects and many other subtle finger functions. Nails are used for decoration and sexual attraction in women, for scratching in response to pruritus and, occasionally, as weapons of aggression. Finger nails typically cover approximately one-seventh of the dorsal surface, while on the great toe the nail may cover up to 50% of the dorsum of the digit.

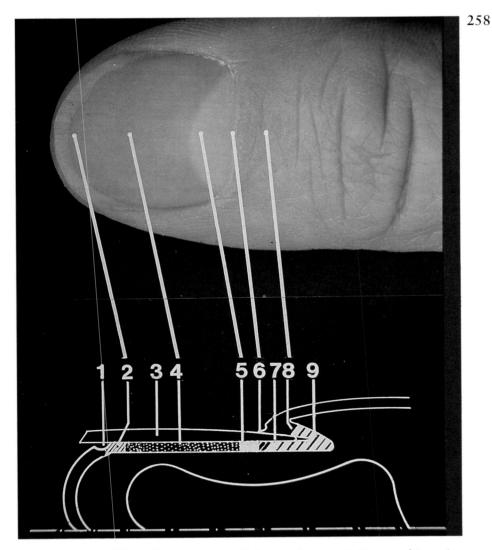

258

258 Anatomy of the nail apparatus: 1. Subungual space. 2. Hyponychium. 3. Nail plate. 4. Nail bed. 5. Distal margin of lunula. 6. Cuticle. 7. Ungual cul de sac (generating the nail plate from the matrix). 8. Proximal nail fold. 9. Nail matrix.

Configuration disorders of nails

Clubbing

The distal end of the digit is bulbous (i.e. club-shaped) with the finger nail hypercurved in longitudinal and transverse planes. The nail base (matrix area) may be easily rocked by pressing gently on its distal end; the movement can be felt by placing a finger over the proximal nail fold of the affected nail. Viewed from the side, the angle between the proximal nail fold and the proximal part of the nail plate is flatter than normal and may exceed 180 degrees.

Schamroth's window test is very helpful clinically (**261, 262**). The nails and dorsal phalangeal joints of the thumbs are placed into apposition. Normally a closed, lozenge-shaped gap results, whereas in clubbing there is a V-shaped gap, widening at the top.

Clubbing is probably caused by hypervascularity and the opening up of many anastomotic channels.

259

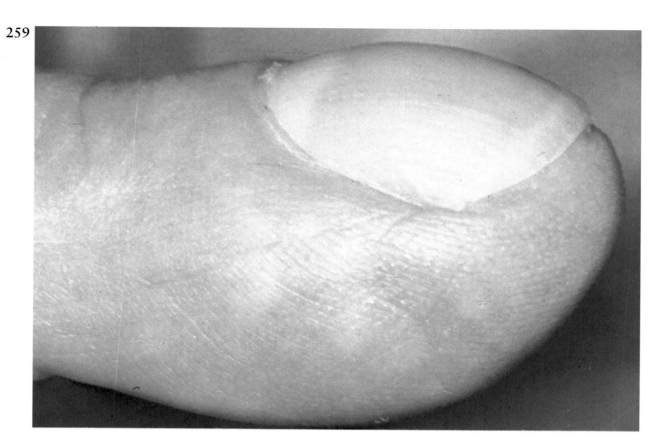

259 Clubbing.

Causes of clubbing

Finger nail clubbing can result from disorders of several systems:

- Chest disease, e.g. bronchiectasis, bronchial carcinoma.
- Cardiovascular disease, e.g. cyanotic congenital heart disease, subacute bacterial endocarditis.
- Liver disease, e.g. hepatic cirrhosis.

260 Clubbing.

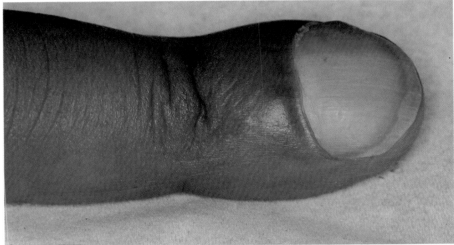

260

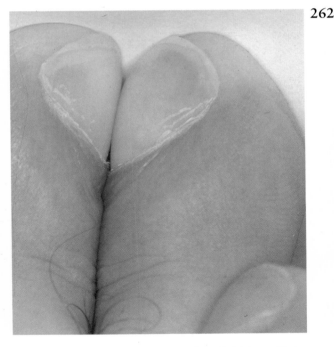

261

262

261 Schamroth's window test for clubbing. Normal nails show an enclosed gap when the thumbs are opposed.

262 Schamroth's window test for clubbing. Clubbed nails show a V-shaped gap at the top when the thumbs are opposed.

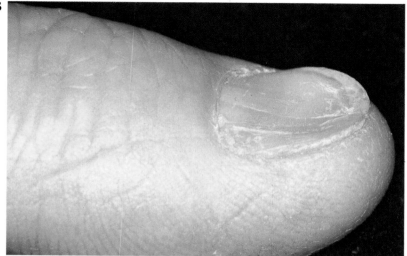

263 **Koilonychia** is the name given to concave or spoon-shaped nail plates. The nail plate itself may be thinned, thickened or normal. There is a form of congenital koilonychia in early infancy that lasts only a few months. Acquired koilonychia may arise from a number of causes: cardiological, haematological (especially iron deficiency anaemia), endocrine, occupational and traumatic.

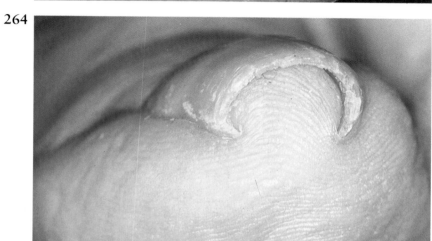

264 **Transverse overcurvature of hallux nails.** The overcurvature in this often hereditary disorder can cause trauma to the lateral nail folds and the development of infection and swelling, the so-called ingrowing toe nails. Overcurvature is a common feature of yellow nail syndrome, where it involves all the digits.

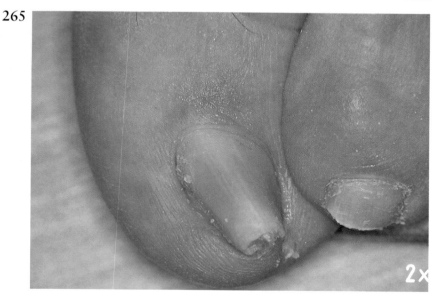

265 **Trumpet nail (pincer nail):** a more extreme example of overcurvature of the nails, with progressive lateral compression of the subungual tissue.

266 Brachyonychia, a defect that usually affects one or both thumbs, is also called racquet nail and is often the result of an inherited short distal phalanx caused by early obliteration of the epiphyseal line. It can also be acquired, e.g. in hyperparathyroidism.

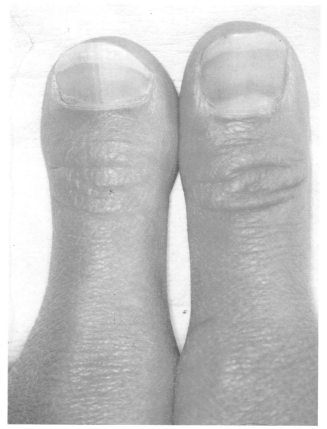

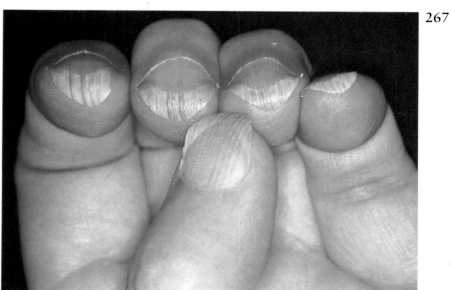

267 Parrot beak nails: longitudinal hypercurvature of the nails.

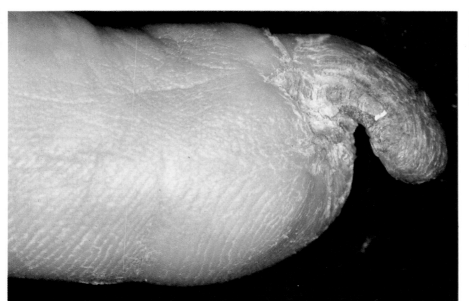

268 Claw-like nail. The shape of this nail has resulted from a shortening of the distal bony phalanx; it is sometimes seen physiologically in the fifth toe nail.

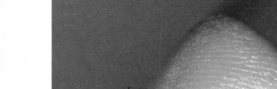

269 Micronychia can be congenital or acquired. A very small nail on the fifth toe is shown, due to continuous pressure from shoes.

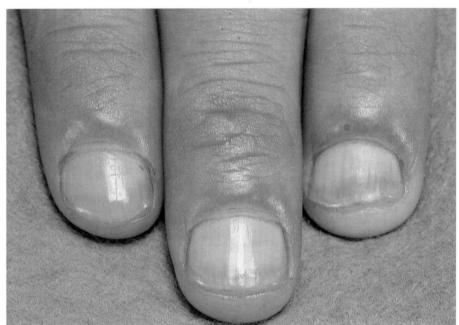

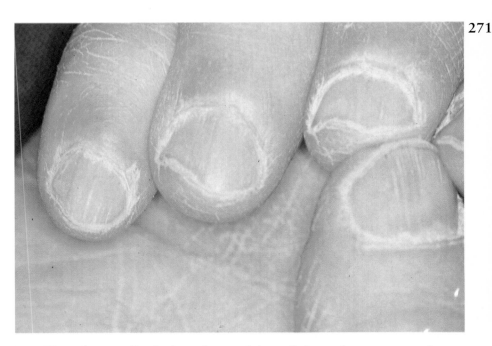

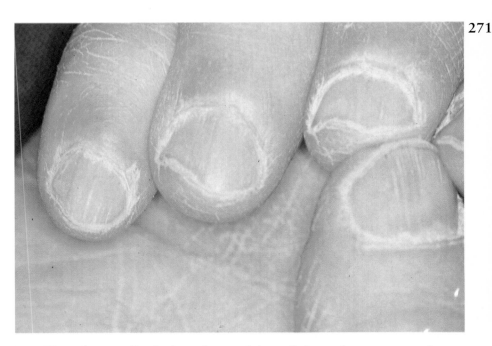

270 Burnished nails. The high burnish or polish on the nails comes about through friction and rubbing against soft material, either in manicuring or due to rubbing the skin with the nail plates. They are often seen in association with very itchy skin disorders, such as chronic atopic dermatitis and advanced mycosis fungoides, and may eventuate in worn down nails.

271 Worn down nails: the lateral part of the nail shows the most wear. Apart from chronic scratching, nails may be worn down in people occupied in heavy manual labour (*usure des ongles*).

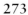

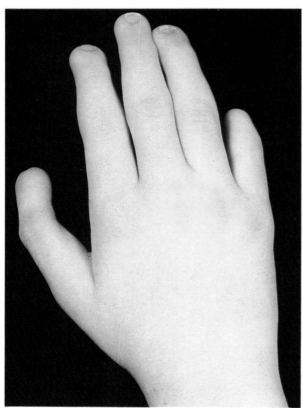

272 Anonychia (see also **421**). The complete absence of one or more nails is a rare congenital disorder associated with absence or hypoplasia of the distal bony phalanx.

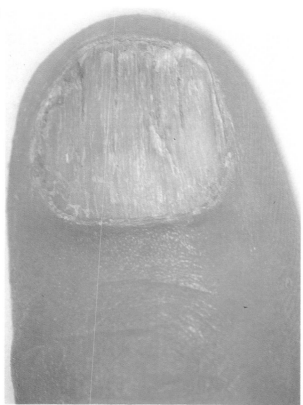

273 Onychoatrophy: there is reduction in size and thickness of the nail plate, often with splitting and fragmentation of the nail. It may be congenital or acquired. Lichen planus is frequently a cause, resulting in atrophy with subsequent scarring and pterygium formation.

274 Hypertrophy of the nails (pachyonychia, ony-chauxis) and **294**, subungual hyperkeratosis. There is hyperkeratosis of the nail bed, the causes of which may be congenital, vascular impairment, trauma, or ageing. It may result from thickening of the nail plate or of the subungual tissues. Hyperplasia of the distal subungual epithelium results in a mass of keratin, variably soft and friable, which pushes the free end of the nail upwards. It is commonly found in inflammatory conditions, e.g. psoriasis, eczema and ringworm fungal infections. A similar appearance is sometimes seen in subungual viral warts, lichen planus and Darier's disease.

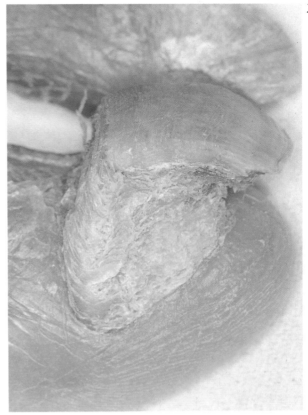

275 Onychogryphosis: usually acquired as a result of self neglect or mental illness. Pressure from footwear causes the untrimmed nail to grow unevenly, producing thickened, curly and ridged nails. The hallux nails are the most likely to be affected. There is a hereditary form, in which all the toe nails and even the finger nails are involved. (Courtesy Prof. Claire Beylot.)

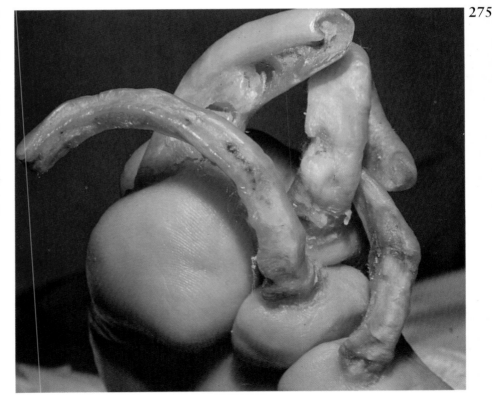

Nail surface changes

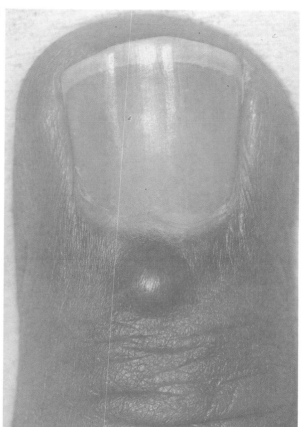

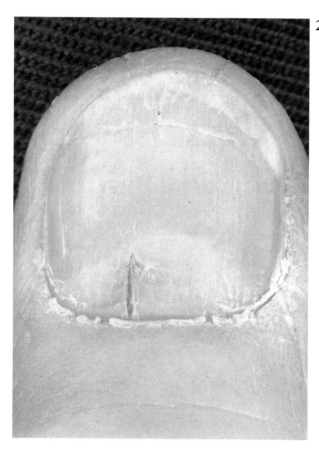

276 Longitudinal grooves may be multiple and develop physiologically with increasing age, or single and the result of pressure on the matrix from a tumour or cystic lesion. **276** shows a groove caused by a myxoid cyst of the proximal nail fold.

277–279 Median nail dystrophy. In this disorder there is a defect of the middle part of the nail, starting proximally (**277**) and extending distally to involve the whole nail plate (**278**). Chevron-shaped cracks may extend laterally from the defect. The thumb nails are most commonly affected. The cause is unknown, but probably traumatic (pressure), and there is often a particularly large lunula. The condition is self-limiting and eventually resolves, but relapses are common. **279** shows a resolving lesion.

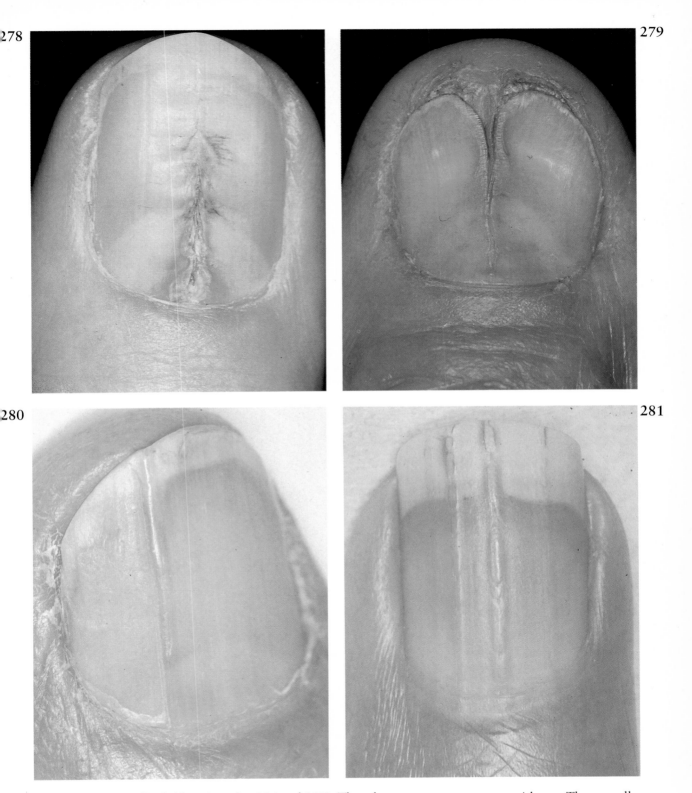

280, 281 Longitudinal ridges (see also **316** and **317**). These become more numerous with age. They usually extend the whole length of the nail, but may be interrupted at regular intervals, giving a beaded or melted wax appearance.

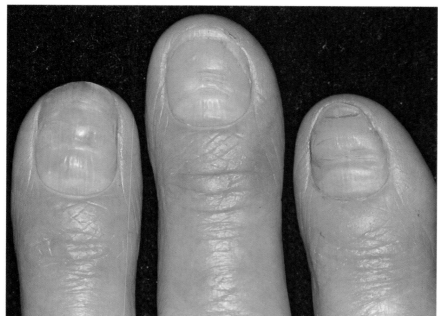

282, 283 Beau's lines and transverse grooves. In this condition there are transverse lines and sulci, affecting all or most of the nails, at the same level. The grooves are a retrospective sign of a profound disturbance of the nail matrix, and follow major illness, such as severe infections (pneumonia, peritonitis), and trauma. As the nails grow out the lines pass more distally. It may take 5 to 6 months for a thumb nail to grow out completely, and up to 18 months for a hallux nail. From the position of the groove it is often possible to estimate when the severe illness occurred.

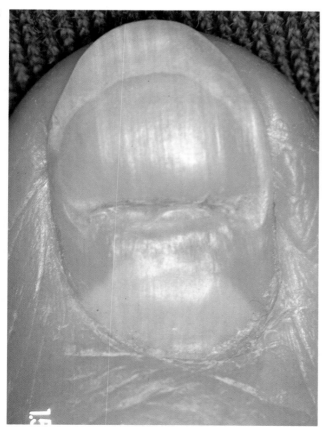

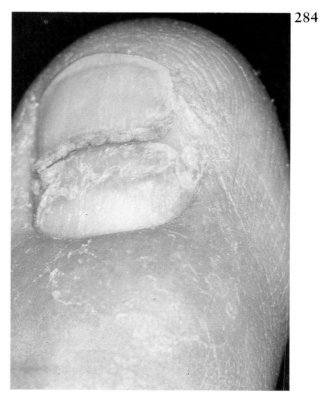

284 If the Beau's lines are very wide there is eventual nail shedding (onychomadesis) of the distal part of the nail (pushed outwards by the newly regenerating nail).

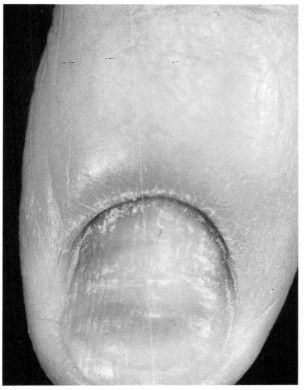

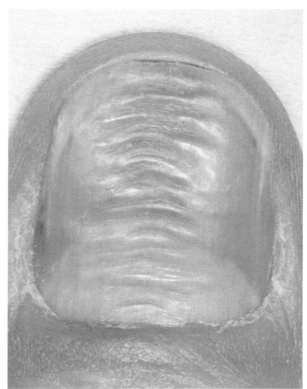

285 Chronic paronychia: there is loss of cuticle and retraction of the nail fold. It is often due to chronic infection by candida albicans and bacteria. The inflammation causes bolstering of the nail folds with secondary nail dystrophy. The problem is often occupational in individuals whose hands are frequently in water (e.g. hairdressers, nurses, laundry workers and food handlers). The nail may be discoloured in its lateral margin. (See also **327, 328, 329.**)

286 Habit tic (washboard thumb nails). There is a central longitudinal irregular groove made up of multiple transverse lines. The pattern is produced by repeated mild retraction injury to the posterior nail fold, usually from the adjacent index finger nail.

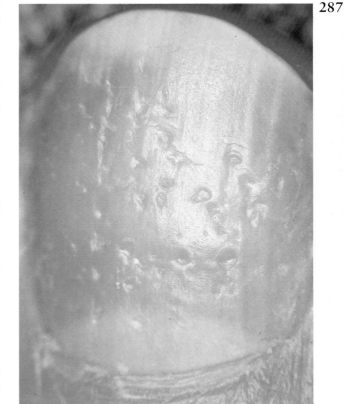

287 Pitting. Pits develop as a result of a transient punctate disturbance of the nail matrix. They may be few or profuse, patterned or random. Pitting is most commonly found in psoriasis, but it can also be a feature of alopecia areata and eczema.

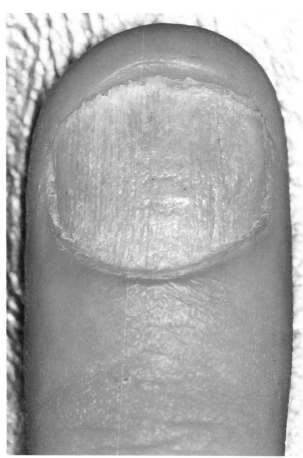

288 Trachyonychia (rough nails, sandpapered nails): the nail has a rough surface, is grey and opaque, and may show splitting at the free margin. It can also be isolated to one or several nails, or may be part of a 20-nail dystrophy as found in alopecia areata or lichen planus. Sometimes the condition appears unassociated with any other skin disorder.

289 Lamellar nail splitting (onychoschizia lamellina). There is splitting into layers of the free margin of the nail. The index and middle finger nails are most often affected, a sign of repeated microtrauma. Sometimes there is a background of poor circulation, but most often the condition is promoted by excessive water immersion.

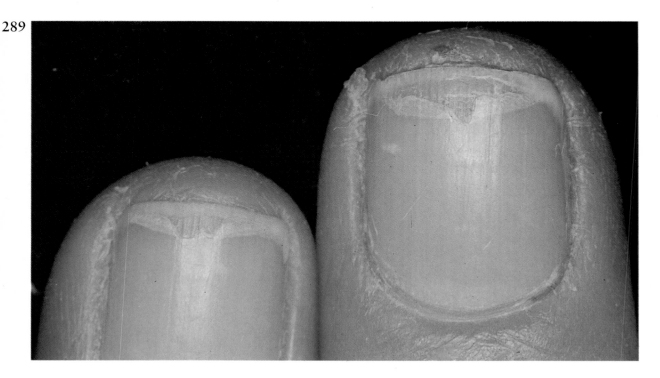

Disorders of the nail plate and associated soft tissue

Pterygium

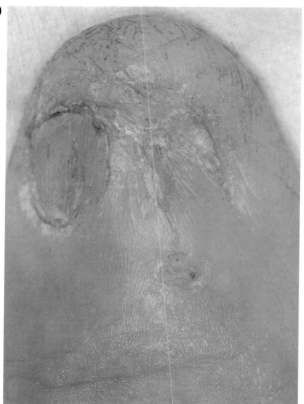

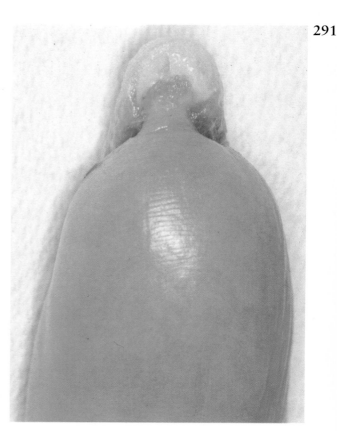

290 Dorsal pterygium: thinning of the posterior nail fold occurs, with adherence to the matrix and triangular extension of the cuticle distally over the nail plate. The nail is gradually eroded at this point and becomes divided into two fragments. The end result can be total loss of nail (sometimes with lateral remnants) and nail bed scarring. This pattern is most commonly seen in lichen planus, but occurs also in digital ischaemia, dystrophic bullous disorders, after radiotherapy, and following trauma.

291 Ventral pterygium (pterygium inversum unguis). In this condition, affecting the finger nails, there is distal extension of the hyponychium, which adheres to the underside of the nail, obliterating the distal groove. It occurs in conditions of scarring of the dermis in the distal groove area, particularly in Raynaud's phenomenon as found in some cases of systemic sclerosis and systemic lupus erythematosus. Rarer causes are causalgia of the median nerve and trauma, and there is a congenital painful familial variety.

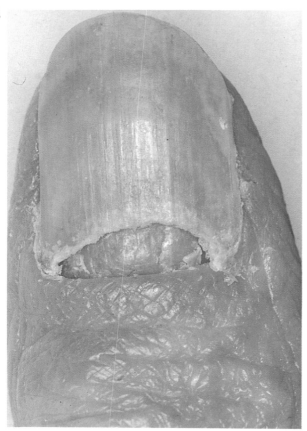

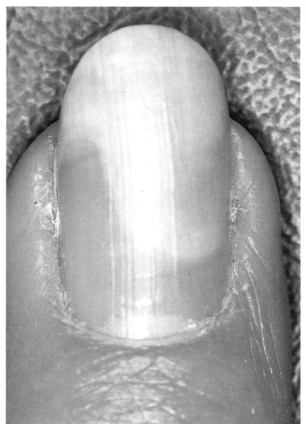

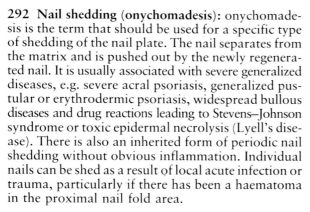

292 Nail shedding (onychomadesis): onychomadesis is the term that should be used for a specific type of shedding of the nail plate. The nail separates from the matrix and is pushed out by the newly regenerated nail. It is usually associated with severe generalized diseases, e.g. severe acral psoriasis, generalized pustular or erythrodermic psoriasis, widespread bullous diseases and drug reactions leading to Stevens–Johnson syndrome or toxic epidermal necrolysis (Lyell's disease). There is also an inherited form of periodic nail shedding without obvious inflammation. Individual nails can be shed as a result of local acute infection or trauma, particularly if there has been a haematoma in the proximal nail fold area.

293 Onycholysis, one of the commonest forms of nail dystrophy, is the detachment of the nail bed at its distal end and/or its lateral attachments. The separation may be partial, or complete and regular — half-moon shaped — or irregular in pattern. Usually some of the nails are spared. It is usually symptomless. The finger nails show onycholysis particularly in psoriasis (**336**) and trauma, less frequently in ringworm fungal infection, candida infection, photo-onycholysis and poor peripheral circulation. In many patients no cause for the onycholysis is found (idiopathic type). Toe nails (particularly hallux nails) produce onycholysis in ringworm fungal infection, and more often with repeated microtrauma and pressure, or from over-riding of the second toe.

Changes in the consistency of the nail plate

- Hard nails (294): Pachyonychia congenita **422, 423**; yellow nail syndrome (367).
- Soft nails: most commonly due to occupational exposure to water and chemicals, e.g. acids and alkalis; can also occur in disease,

e.g. chronic arthritis, myxoedema and digital ischaemia.
- Brittle nails: usually due to over-immersion in hot water, soap, detergents and solvents.

294 Hard nails.

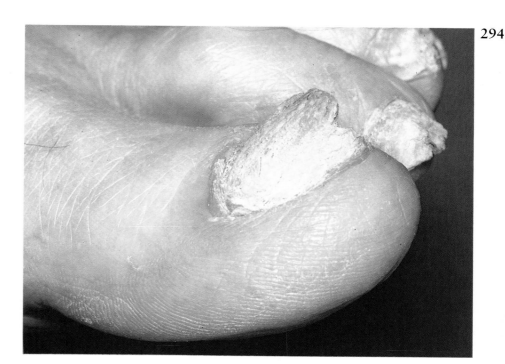

294

295 Brittle nails.

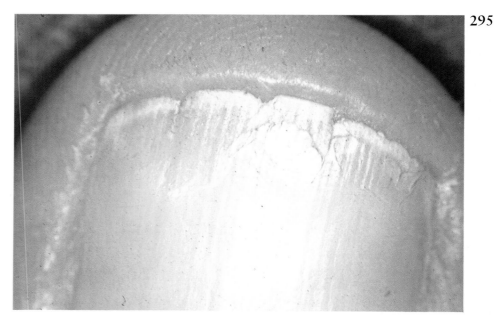

295

Colour changes in nails

The discoloration may be on the surface of the nail plate, within the nail plate, or in the nail bed.

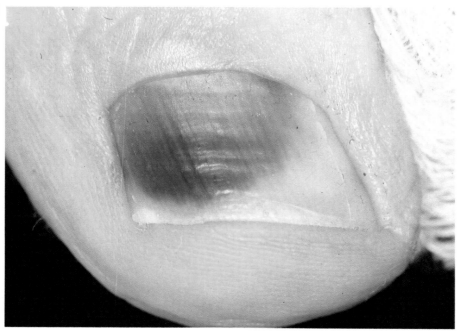

296 Subungual haematoma of hallux.

Causes of nail discoloration:

- Exogenous causes: topical medicaments and dyes, tobacco, occupational chemical contact, infection with fungi, yeast or bacteria (blue-black colour is usually caused by *Pseudomonas pyocyanea* either on its own or in association with other infection, especially candida).
- Systemic drugs and chemicals.
- Dermatological conditions. Longitudinal brown bands are seen in melanocytic hyperplasia, naevi, malignant melanoma, trauma (especially in black people) and sometimes in lichen planus.
- Systemic infections cause a variety of rarely seen changes; perhaps the commonest is the presence of brown splinter haemorrhages in subacute bacterial endocarditis.
- Non-infective systemic conditions. Yellow nail syndrome produces yellowing of the nails only (367). Cardiac failure and peripheral vascular insufficiency cause blue nails and gangrene causes blackening of the whole digit. Reddish lunules are sometimes seen in cardiac failure, cirrhosis, rheumatoid arthritis, psoriasis and alopecia areata.

White nails (apparent leukonychia) sparing the distal portion are seen in hepatic cirrhosis. In chronic renal disease the pattern is of the half-and-half nail, where the proximal half is white and the distal half is pink, sometimes resembling a crescent.

297 *Pseudomonas pyocyanea* infection of the nail.

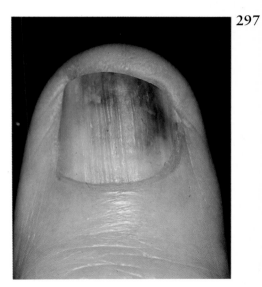

298 Copper sulphate soaks have produced blue nails.

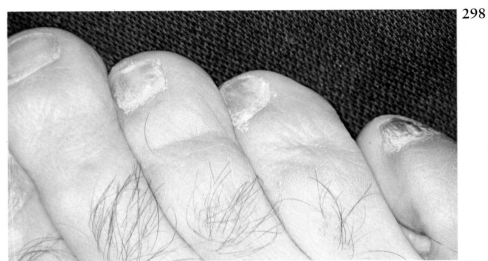

299 Iodine staining: the outgrowing arc parallel to the curve of the proximal nail fold is characteristic of an exogenous cause.

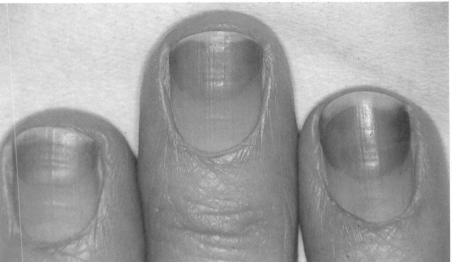

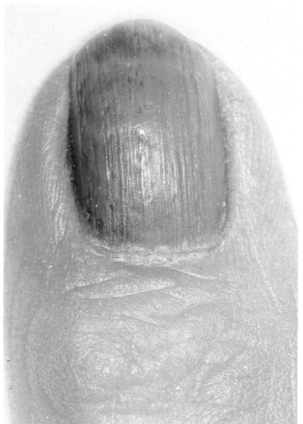

300 Tobacco staining. The familiar type of brown staining resulting from heavy cigarette smoking shown here must be distinguished from other forms of nail discoloration. The nail plate and one lateral nail fold are heavily stained.

Systemic drugs and chemicals: antimalarials (blue or purple tints) (see 405).

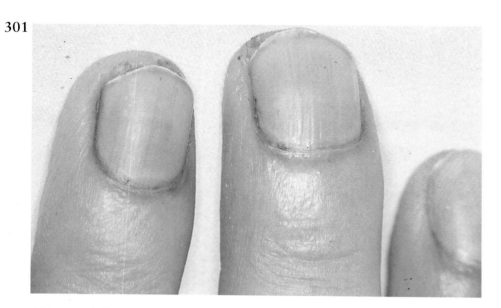

301 Non-infective systemic conditions: jaundice affecting distal fingers and nail beds.

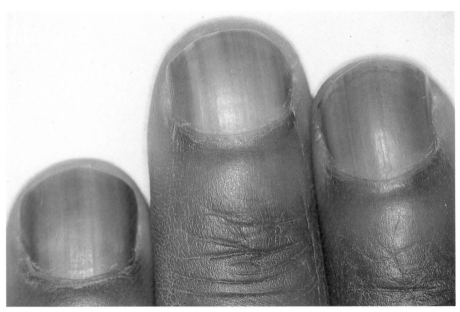

302 Longitudinal dyschromic bands (longitudinal melanonychia). Dark bands are common in black individuals and mostly occur for no apparent reason. However, in Caucasians they may indicate a significant disorder such as malignant melanoma, Addison's disease, or vitamin B12 deficiency. White and red longitudinal bands occurring together are pathognomonic of Darier's disease (**360**).

Leukonychia

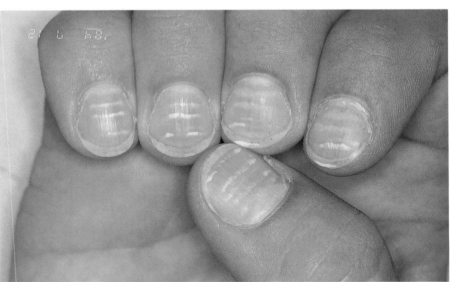

303 Transverse striate leukonychia. One or more nails show transverse white bands. These lines arise from repeated minor trauma to the nail matrix, often from manicuring and pushing back cuticles or from liquid nitrogen therapy for periungual viral warts. More rarely, white bands in most or all nails are caused by a severe systemic illness and have the same significance as Beau's lines and are present at the same level on several nails (**282-284**).

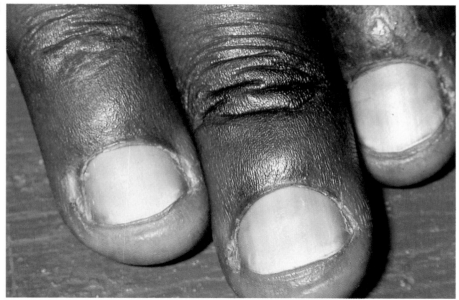

304 'True' total leukonychia. This is a rare hereditary form of leukonychia affecting all the nails. Pseudoleukonychia is the term used for superficially friable white nails due to fungal infection or the granulation of nail keratin resulting from applications of fresh coats of varnish on top of old, worn varnish, for several weeks in succession.

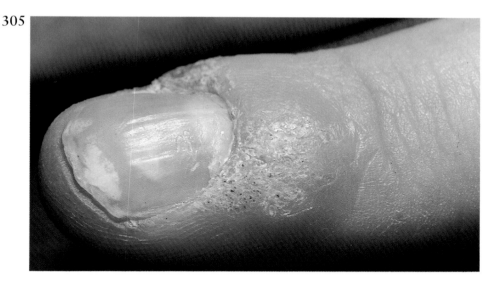

305 Leukonychia resulting from repeated liquid nitrogen treatment to a viral wart of the nail fold.

Half-and-half nail in uraemia (see 370). The proximal area is pale with indiscernible lunula and the distal area is pink.

The nail in childhood and old age

306 Normal child's nail. Physiological oblique ridges are sometimes seen.

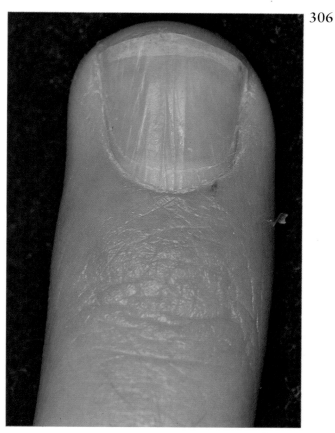

307 Infantile koilonychia. Koilonychia of the hallux nail is not rare, but physiologically in infants it is a temporary phenomenon.

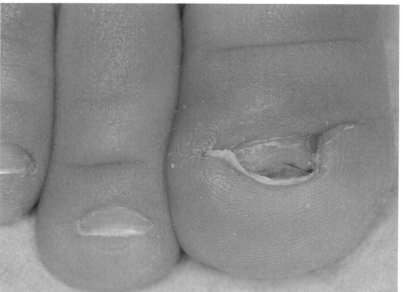

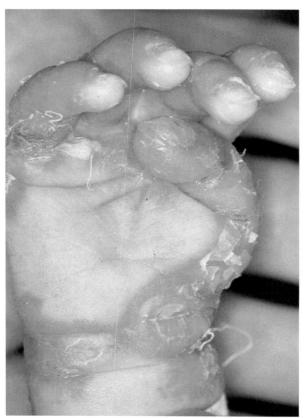

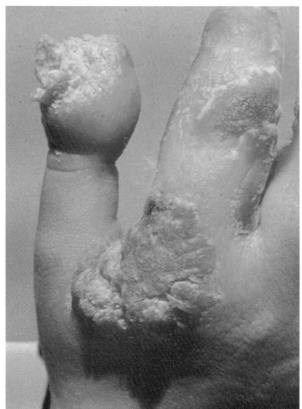

308 Zinc deficiency: there are periungual eczematous changes with secondary nail dystrophy. In later life this syndrome may be associated with prolonged parenteral nutrition.

309 Candida infection. In children, nail plate infection with candida is a sign of chronic mucocutaneous candidiasis, a disorder associated with immunological deficiency and low serum iron.

310 Thumb sucking is a habit common in children and causes maceration of the periungual skin and sometimes nail plate changes, usually with candida infection.

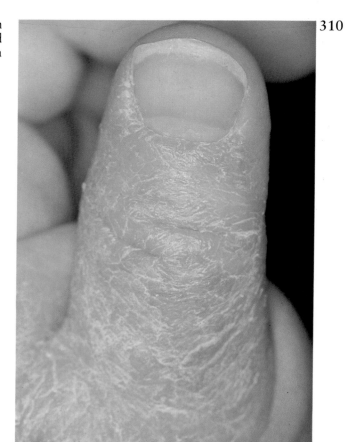

311 Congenital malalignment of the hallux nail. In this condition the axis of the nail plate is deviated laterally. It may be complicated by ingrowing toenail and paronychia. It is susceptible to surgical correction.

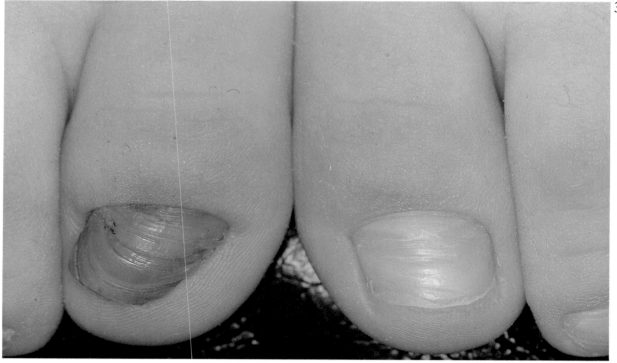

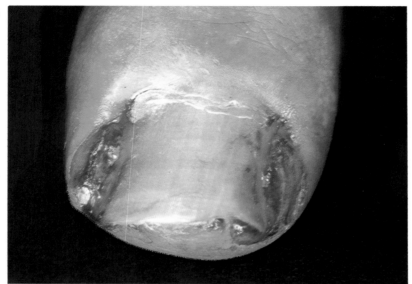

312 Ingrowing toenail, juvenile type. The lateral margin of the nail is growing into the nail fold and external pressure has caused trauma and paronychia. If neglected, the disability becomes severe and repeated episodes occur.

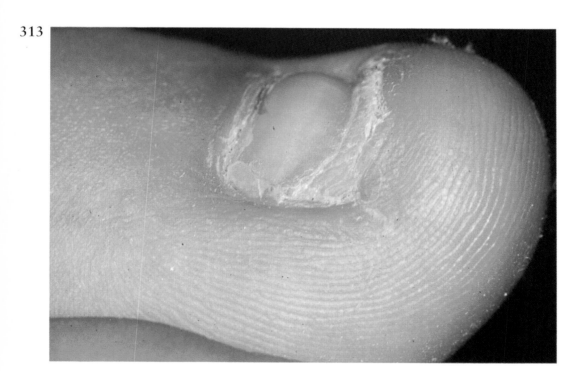

313 Ingrowing toenail, distal embedded type (tennis toe): this follows shedding or therapeutic avulsion of the hallux nail. The new nail becomes embedded in distal pulp tissue that has become heaped up.

314 Childhood psoriasis. Oblique ridging and pitting is shown. Sometimes isolated nail dystrophy is the first sign of childhood psoriasis, with classical plaques appearing after a number of years.

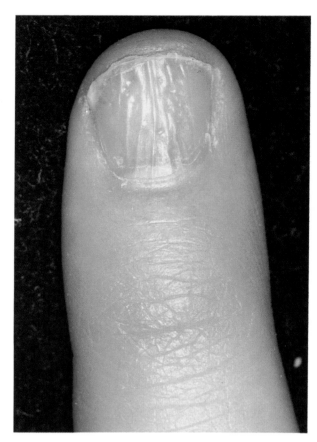

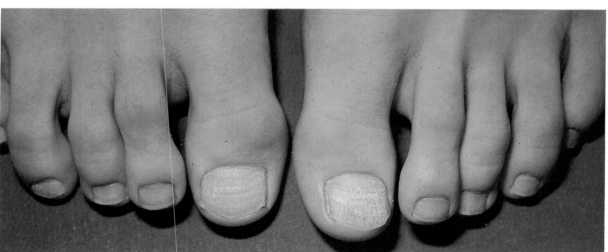

315 Twenty nail dystrophy is the term used for dystrophy of all the finger and toe nails, usually in infants or young children, in which the cause is unknown. The nails are uniformly and simultaneously affected with excess longitudinal ridging and loss of lustre. It is probably best regarded as a physical sign with numerous causes, since many examples are later diagnosed as lichen planus, alopecia areata or psoriasis. Nail biopsy is helpful for the diagnosis of lichen planus.

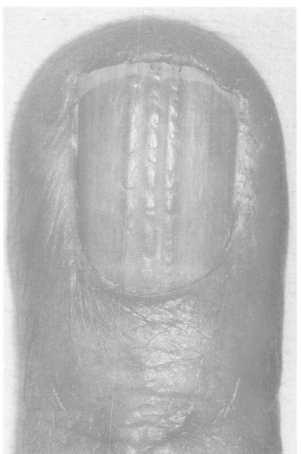
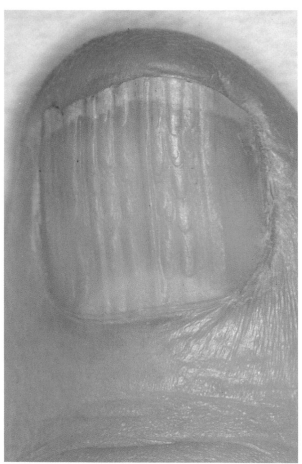

316, 317 Longitudinal ridging increases with age. The ridges may be thin and regular along their length, or they may be beaded, or interrupted like a string of sausages. In the elderly the nail thickness is rather variable, but the finger nails tend to be soft and fragile, the free margins being liable to split longitudinally or into layers. Toe nails tend to be hypertrophic from fungal infection, trauma or pressure from shoes. The incidence of infection by moulds increases with age.

Fungal and other infections of the nails

318 Ringworm fungal infection of the finger nails. The distal parts of several nails show irregular white thickening and onycholysis. The proximal part of the nails is an orange-red colour. The organism was shown to be *Trichophyton rubrum*, an infection usually unilateral when it affects the hands and bilateral on the feet (one-hand-two-feet syndrome). Fungal infection of the nails can be caused by dermatophytes, *Candida* species or moulds.

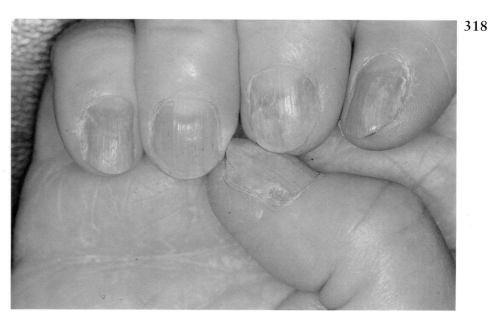

319 Hallux nail ringworm infection. There is distal thickening and onycholysis.

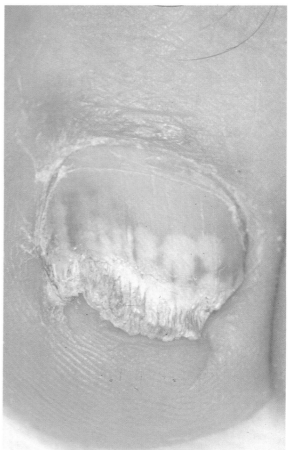

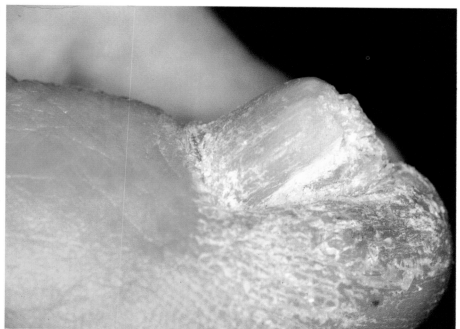

320 Ringworm fungal infection in psoriasis. It is not uncommon for hallux nails to show co-existing psoriatic hypertrophy and ringworm infection, whereas this combination is rare in finger nails.

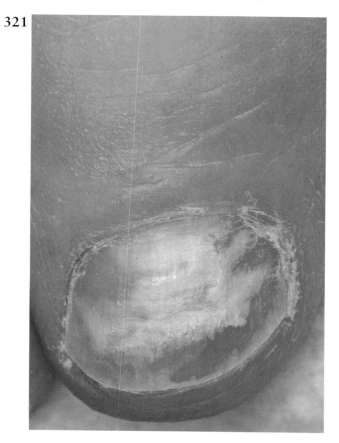

321 Proximal subungual onychomycosis. In this disorder the infection starts proximally in the ventral part of the nail.

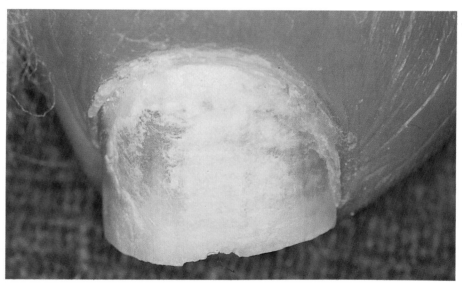

322 White superficial onychomycosis is a pattern of infection usually caused by *Trichophyton mentagrophytes* var. *interdigitale*.

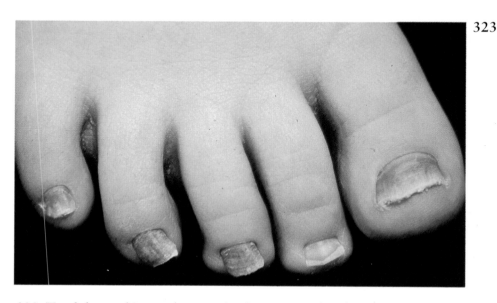

323 Total dystrophic onychomycosis: this term implies that the whole nail is involved in the infection, even though individual nails may be spared. (Courtesy Prof. R. Hay.)

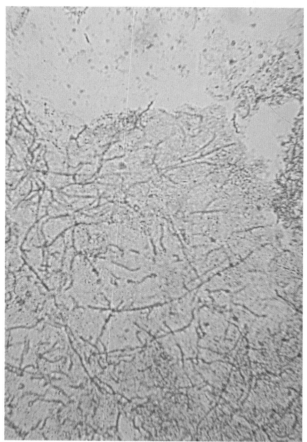

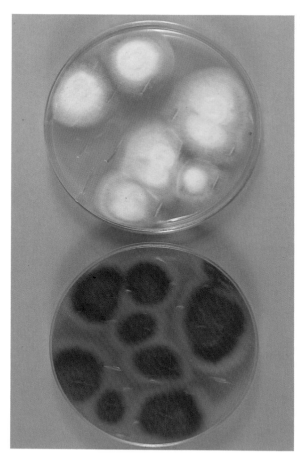

324 Microscopy of scrapings from an infected nail. The friable portion of the nail is scraped or clipped and the material is mounted on a slide in 10% potassium hydroxide solution. Gentle heating hastens clearing for microscopy. The presence of branched fungal mycelium confirms the diagnosis of ringworm. Further specimens are taken for culture.

325 Mycology culture plate showing *Trichophyton rubrum* colonies. The upper plate, viewed from above, shows fluffy white colonies. The lower plate, viewed from below, shows typical brownish-red pigment spreading into the Sabouraud's medium. (Courtesy, Department of Medical Mycology, Institute of Dermatology, London.)

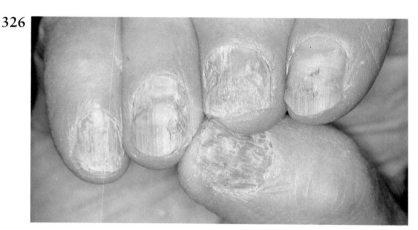

326 Extensive *Candida* infection of the finger nails. This is rare. It occurs in chronic mucocutaneous candidiasis and in other causes of chronic cell-mediated immunodeficiency. It is also a total dystrophic onychomycosis, but primary in contrast to **323**, which is secondary.

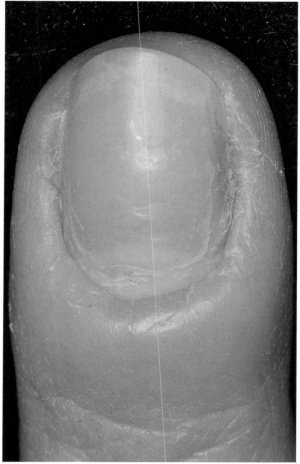

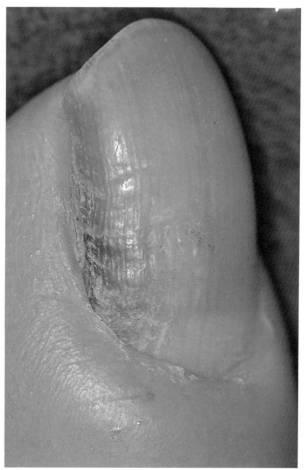

327 Chronic paronychia. An early stage is shown with loss of cuticle and swelling of the posterior and lateral nail folds without nail dystrophy. Intrusion of moisture below the nail fold allows chronic infection with *Candida* and bacteria.

328 Unilateral chronic paronychia: only one lateral nail fold is affected, with transverse grooving of the adjacent part of the nail.

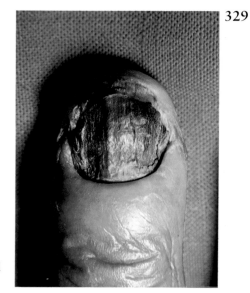

329 Chronic paronychia. Advanced stage showing secondary nail dystrophy.

330

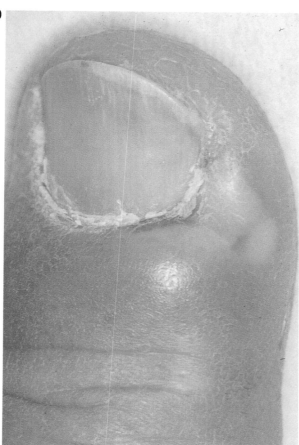

330 Acute bacterial paronychia: a condition caused by *Staphylococcus aureus* or by *Streptococcus pyogenes*. It comes on within a few hours and is intensely painful, throbbing and tender, particularly at night. The infection causes a pustule or abscess. Sometimes there is secondary lymphangitis.

331 *Herpes simplex* (herpetic whitlow). This viral infection is often very painful initially and needs to be differentiated from acute bacterial paronychia. The cluster of vesicles seen here is very typical of the disease. Cytology (Tzanck) smears reveal balloon cells and provide rapid diagnosis. *Herpes simplex* can be recurrent at the same site.

331

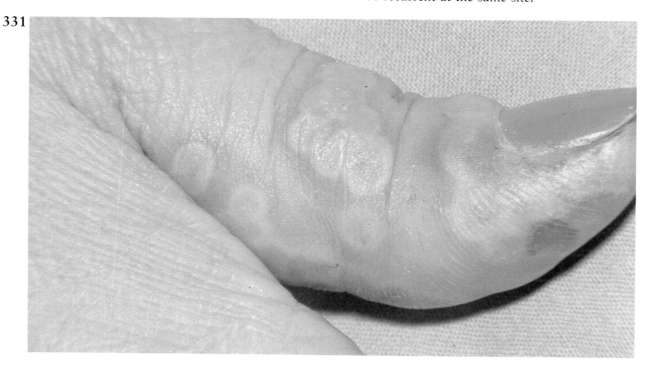

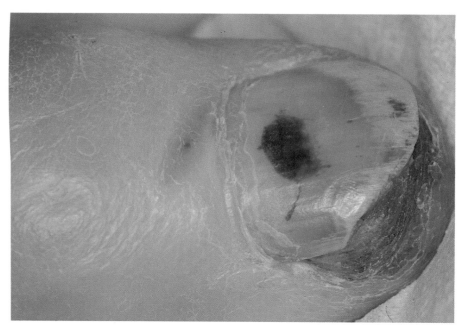

332 Subungual *herpes simplex*: in this form the diagnosis is not obvious unless there is a history of recurrent similar attacks. The diagnosis is proved by viral culture.

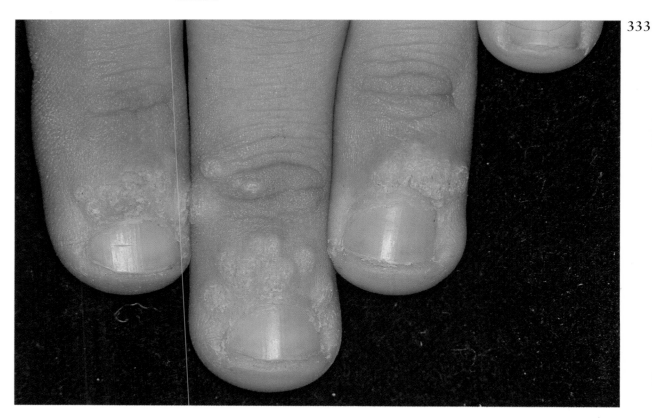

333 Periungual viral warts. These warts on the nail folds are sometimes provoked and spread by biting the nail folds. Viral warts on the lips can co-exist. Surprisingly, nail dystrophy is rare in this condition.

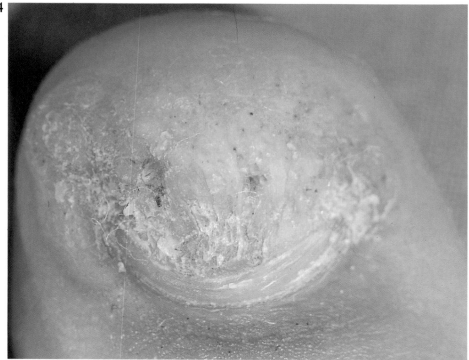

334 Subungual viral wart: here the onycholytic portion of the nail has been trimmed away to reveal a mass of viral wart tissue.

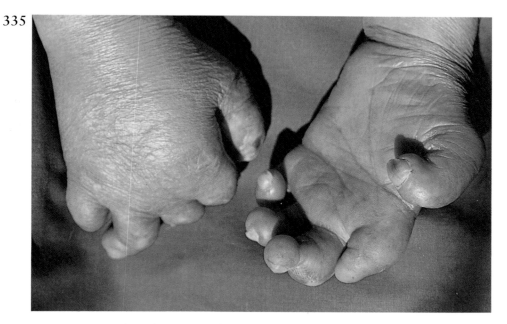

335 Leprosy: the digits are distorted and atrophic secondary to peripheral neuropathy anaesthesia. The nails become clawed and may be lost with atrophic changes in the nail apparatus.

The nail in dermatological diseases

Psoriasis: transient symptoms

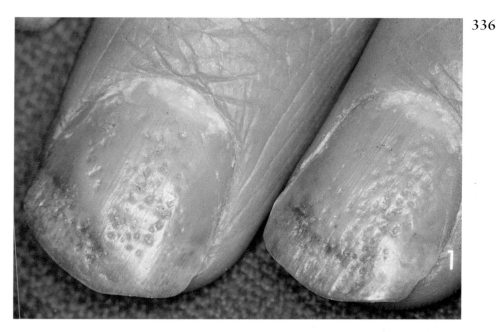

336 Psoriasis, pitting and irregular onycholysis is shown; when sparse, pitting tends to be in longitudinal lines and bands.

337 Psoriasis, with profuse pitting gives a rough look to the nails; the lunulae are partially obscured. Nails of psoriatics grow faster than normal.

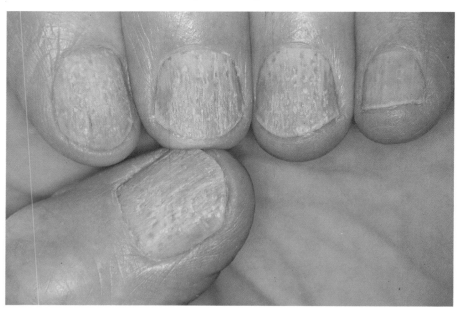

338

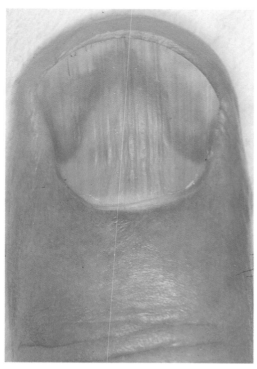

338 Psoriasis onycholysis, typically irregular. There is an orange-red inflamed interface between the normal and the onycholytic area. This is a valuable physical sign of psoriasis.

339

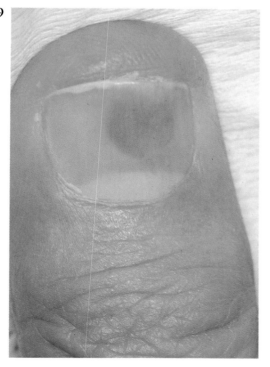

339 Psoriasis: the salmon patch or oil drop sign. One or more orange-pink translucent circular areas appear under the nail plate. This is due to a subungual psoriatic plaque.

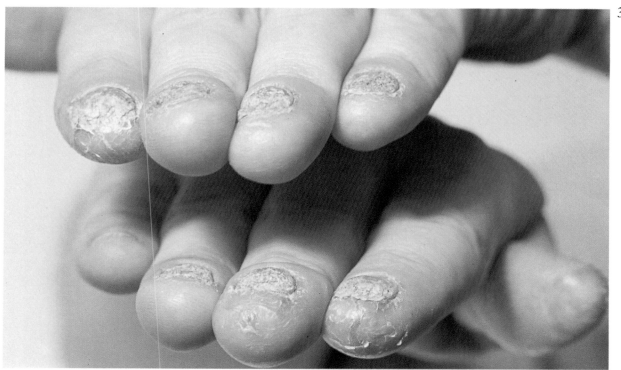

340 Thickened nails in psoriasis.

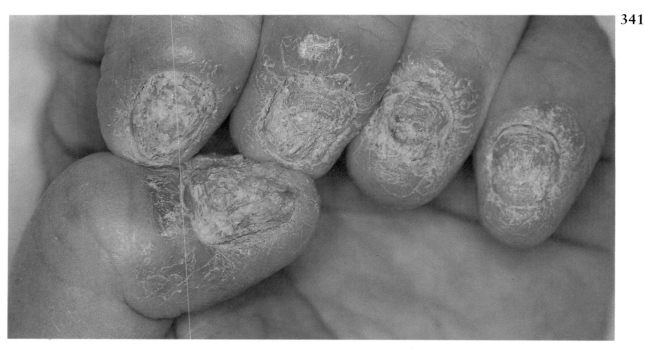

341 **In acral psoriasis the nail dystrophy** is often severe, with irregular thickening of the nail plates.

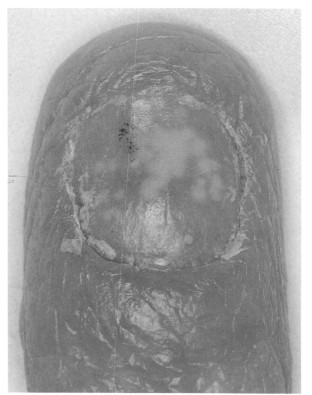

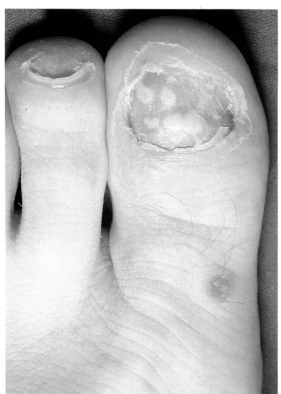

342 Pustular psoriasis: pustules appear in the nail bed. Nail shedding is common.

343 Pustular psoriasis. The nail has been shed.

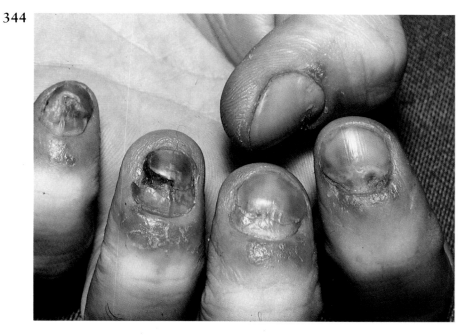

344 Reiter's disease. The skin changes in this disease are best regarded as hyperkeratotic and pustular psoriasis.

Acrokeratosis paraneoplastica (Bazex and Dupré) (see **394**). This condition shows psoriasiform changes of the extremities and nails and affects mainly men over the age of 40. It is associated with malignant disease.

345 Pityriasis rubra pilaris: involvement of the nail bed only. (Matrix has been spared.)

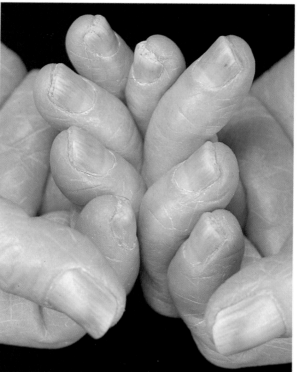

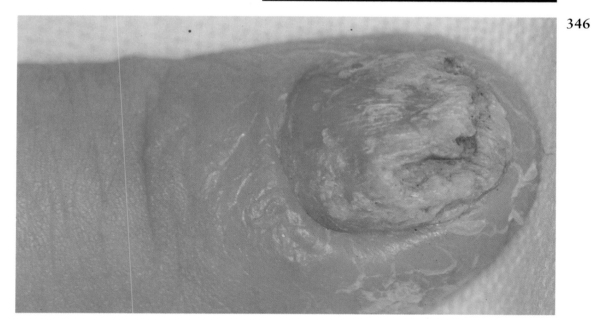

346 Parakeratosis pustulosa. This condition affects prepubertal girls. The initial lesions are very transient pustules of the nail folds followed by inflammation and scaling suggestive of eczema, psoriasis and onychomycosis. The nails may show pitting, fragility, scaling and subungual hyperkeratosis. Most evolve as psoriasis.

347

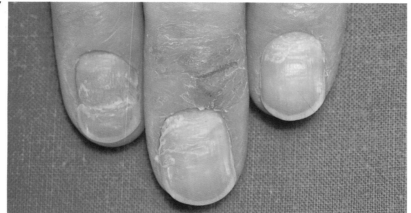

347 Eczema of the nail folds often produces transverse nail grooving, roughness and irregularity. The changes can be seen in any form of eczematous dermatitis that affects the fingers, e.g. irritant contact, allergic contact, photosensitive, atopic, discoid and pompholyx types.

348

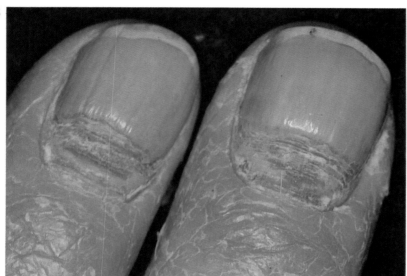

348 This marked nail change occurred acutely in a drug induced photosensitive eczema.

349

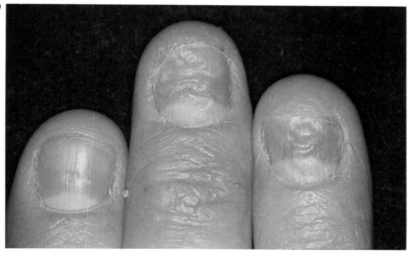

349 Gross nail changes in atopic eczema. Nail changes without eczema of the surrounding tissue suggests isolated matrix involvement.

Lichen planus

About 10% of patients with lichen planus have nail involvement affecting the nail matrix and the nail bed. The changes vary greatly in severity. Usually most of the nails are affected.

350 Lichen planus: the nails show longitudinal fluting with thinning of the nail plate.

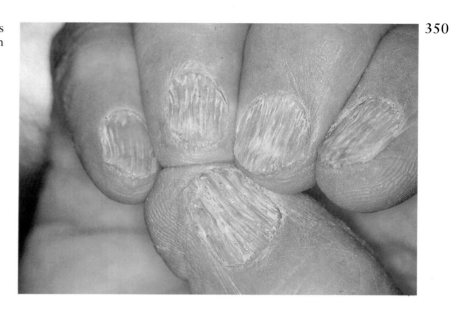

351 Lichen planus: dorsal pterygium. This is a characteristic change of severe lichen planus of the nails (see **352**).

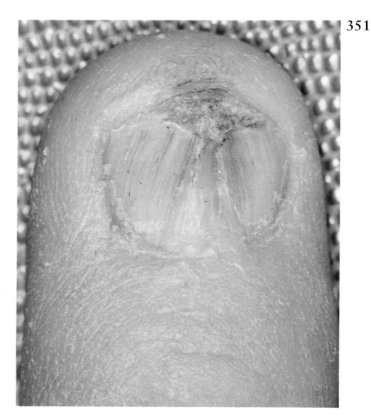

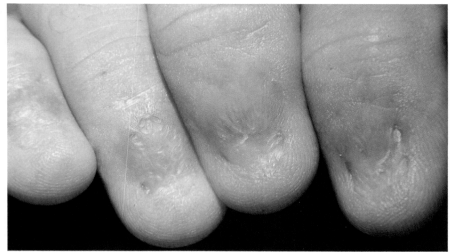

352 Lichen planus: total nail atrophy. The remains of previous pterygium formation are visible.

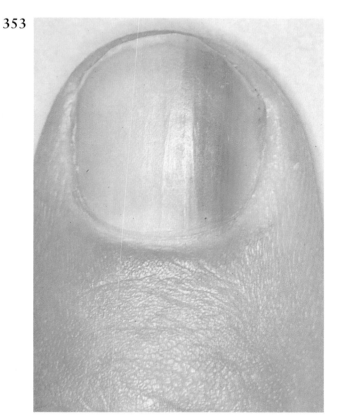

353 Lichen planus. Longitudinal melanonychia is a rare finding which may appear only after the cure of lichen planus.

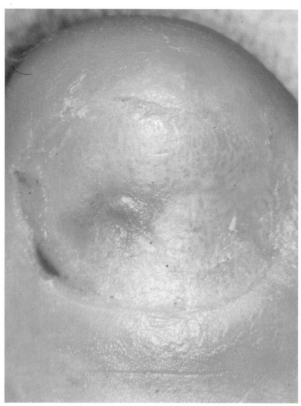

354 Ulcerative lichen planus. The nail apparatus is often severely affected in this acral type of lichen planus.

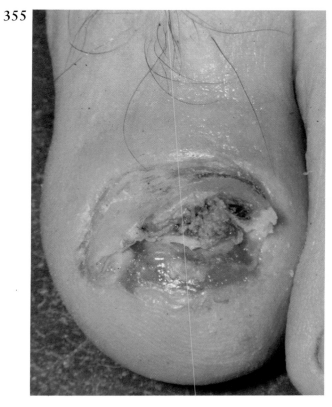

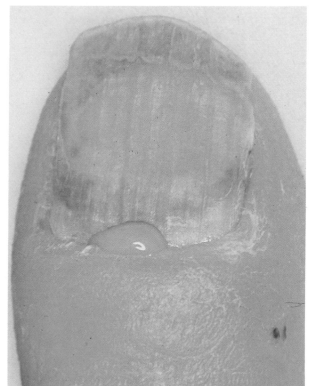

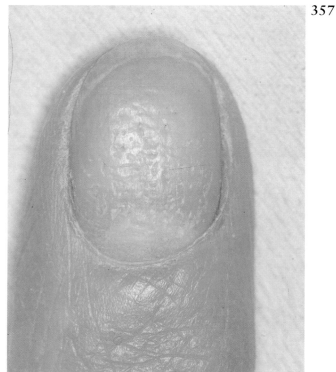

355 Pemphigus: hallux nail, distal erosion and onycholysis. (Courtesy Prof. J. Civatte.)

356 Pemphigus paronychia of the finger nail.

357 Alopecia areata: nail pitting of diffuse and irregular type.

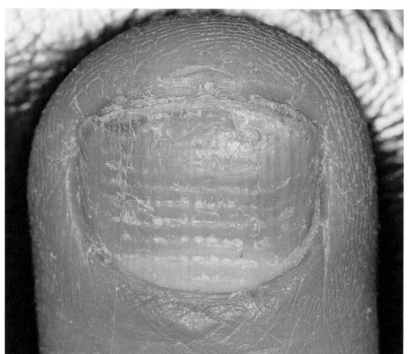

358 Alopecia areata: nail pitting with transverse ripple effect.

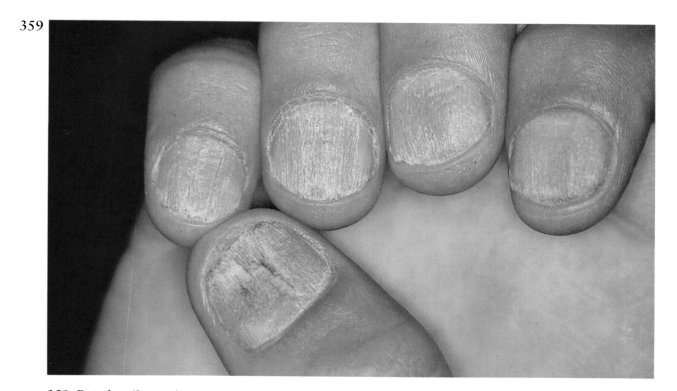

359 Rough nails (trachyonychia). This pattern of roughness and grey opacity of the nail is seen in alopecia areata, lichen planus and psoriasis.

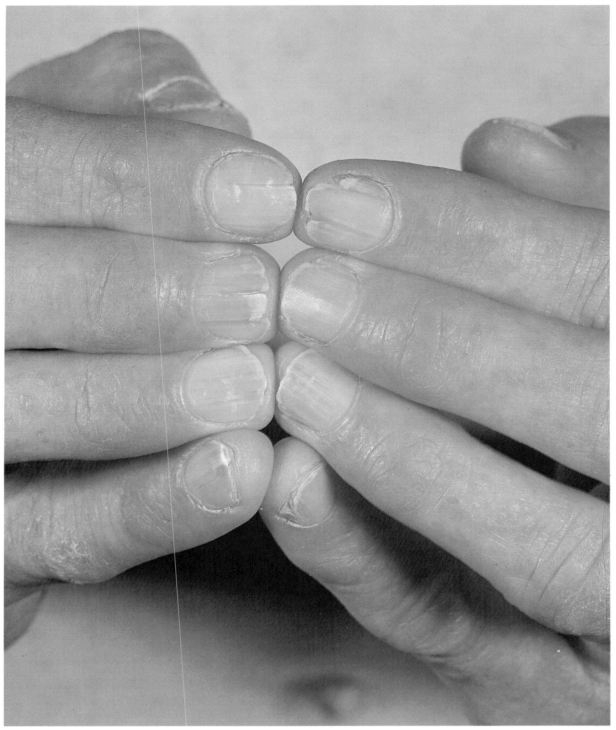

360 Darier's disease: the nail features are distal margin fragility with V-shaped nicks at the free edge, longitudinal ridging, and complete white and red narrow longitudinal bands.

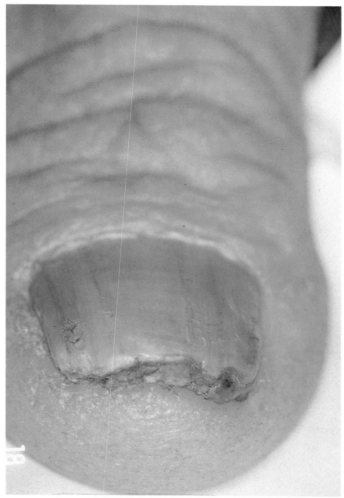

361 Darier's disease: subungual thickening.

The nail in systemic diseases

362 Clubbing in a child with cyanotic congenital heart disease.

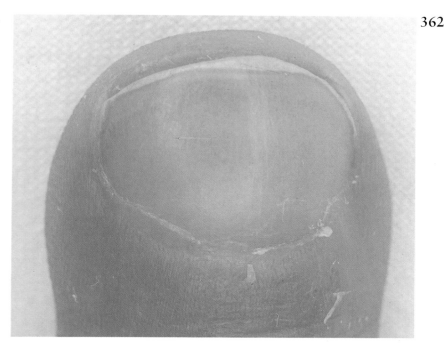

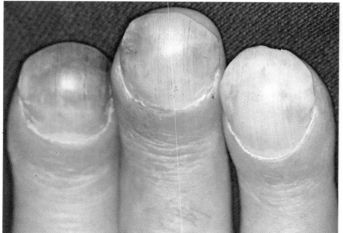

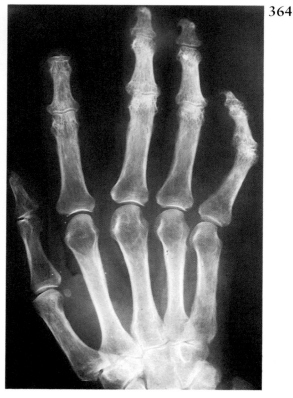

363, 364 Clubbing in pachydermoperiostosis and hypertrophic pulmonary osteoarthropathy. The clinical appearance of the fingers is similar in the two disorders. Pachydermoperiostosis starts at around puberty. Clubbing of digits and periosteal new bone formation (304) are associated with thickening and furrowing of the scalp and face. In hypertrophic pulmonary osteoarthropathy there is inflammatory arthropathy, especially in the lower limbs, and the syndrome is almost invariably associated with a malignant chest tumour.

365

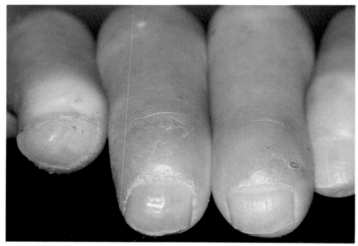

365 Raynaud's disease, due to systemic sclerosis. The nail folds show atrophy, telangiectasia and scarring, with ragged cuticles. The nails are thin and beaked. (See also **388**.)

366

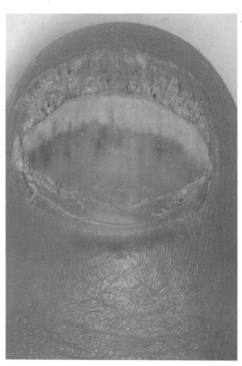

366 Splinter haemorrhages: an important physical sign of septicaemia, particularly subacute bacterial endocarditis. Similar lesions are seen in immune complex vasculitis. Distal splinter haemorrhages are common and usually result from trauma, manual labour and psoriasis.

367

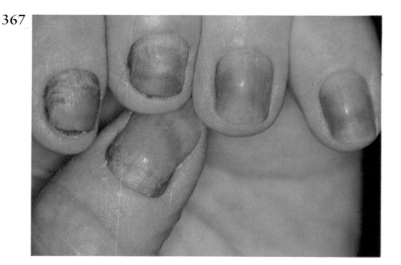

367 Yellow nail syndrome. The nails are yellow, hard and hypercurved transversely with loss of the cuticle and secondary paronychia. Growth is almost arrested and the nails can be further discoloured by *Pseudomonas pyocyanea* infection. The syndrome is associated with a disorder of lymphatics in which there may be lymphoedema of the limbs, pleural effusion and ascites. The nail condition sometimes returns to normal, but relapses are possible.

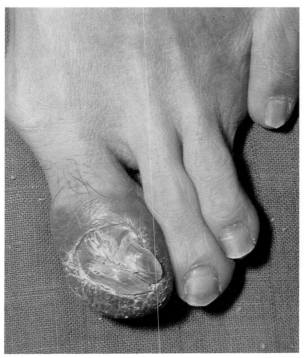

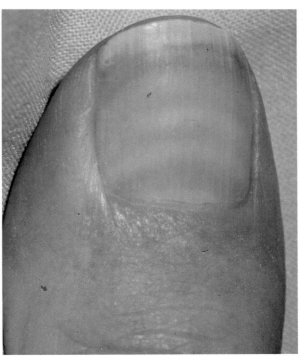

368 Sarcoidosis: the digit is swollen and inflamed and the nail is thickened and fragile. The underlying bony phalanx is always affected.

369 Hypoalbuminaemic white bands (Muehrcke's lines). A pair of transverse white bands are seen, distal to the lunula. They are seen only when the serum albumin falls chronically below 2 gm per 100 ml. The commonest association is the nephrotic syndrome. (Courtesy Dr. K. Thomsen.)

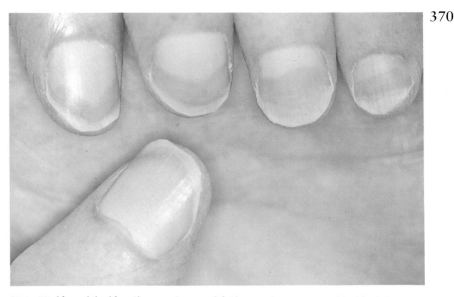

370 Half-and-half nails seen in renal failure. The proximal half of the nail is white and the distal half is pink or pigmented. (Courtesy Dr. K. Thomsen.)

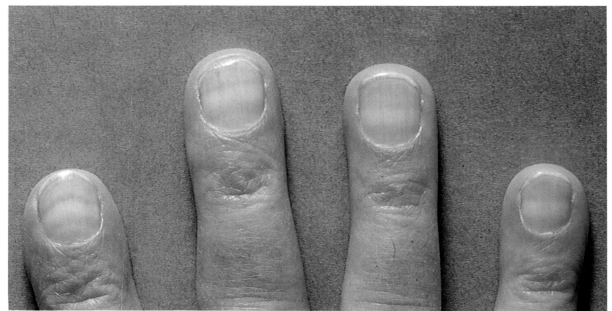

371 Cirrhosis: white nails in hepatocellular disease, resulting either from pallor of the nail beds or from chronic hypoalbuminaemia.

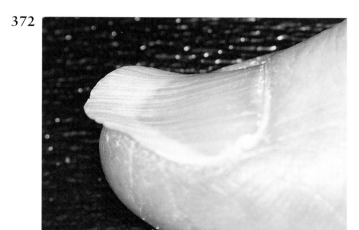

372 Plummer–Vinson syndrome: a syndrome of glossitis, dysphagia and iron deficiency anaemia in which koilonychia (shown here) is found in about half the cases.

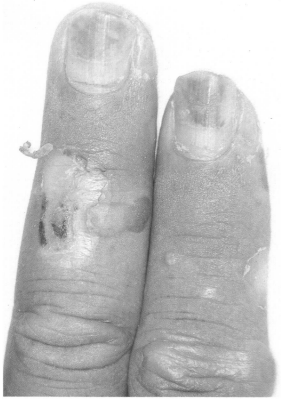

373 Porphyria cutanea tarda. Photo-onycholysis is shown, with blisters and erosions of the dorsal fingers.

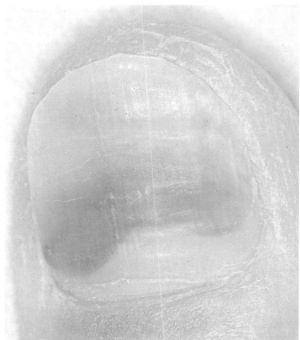

374 Porphyria cutanea tarda: a subungual blister. The greenish colour is due to *Pseudomonas* infection.

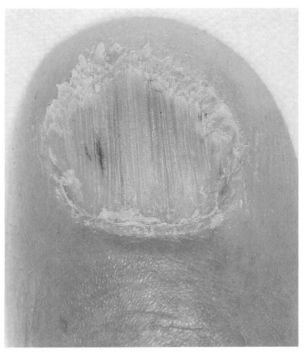

375 Amyloidosis: onychoatrophy, resembling lichen planus.

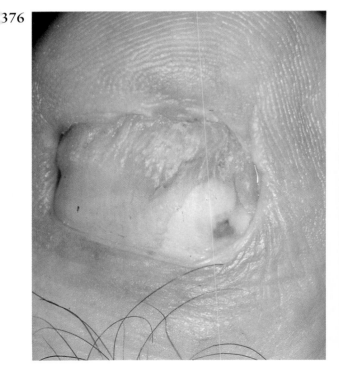

376 Gout. There is nail dystrophy, with a small fistula.

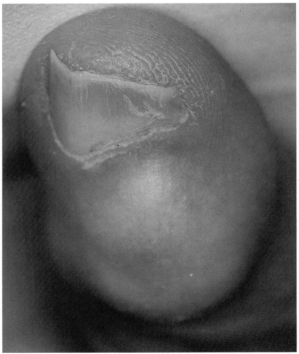

377 Gout. A tophus has encroached on the nail.

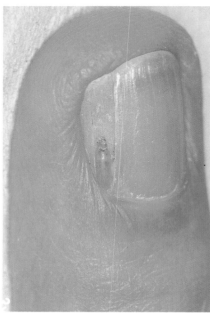

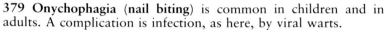

379 Onychophagia (nail biting) is common in children and in adults. A complication is infection, as here, by viral warts.

378 Periungual fibroma (Koenen's tumour) is found in epiloia. Associated features are cerebral tuberose sclerosis, epilepsy, facial adenoma sebaceum, shagreen patches and renal hamartomas. The disorder is inherited as an autosomal dominant. Considerable variation in expression of the disease is seen; sometimes the periungual fibromas are the only sign, appearing at 12 years of age.

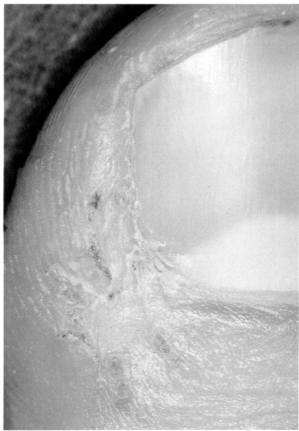

380 Hang nail: a small, tender, partially detached piece of skin from the lateral nail fold. It is usually caused by habit tic picking.

381 Washboard deformity: the thumb nails are here symmetrically affected. There is a wide central groove made up of numerous small transverse grooves. It is caused by repeated self induced trauma to the centre of the posterior nail fold, usually by the adjacent index finger.

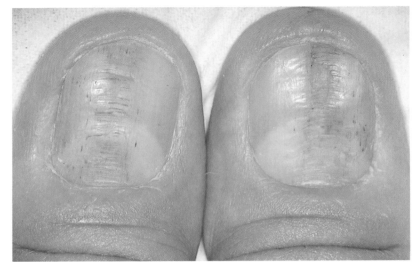
381

382 Onychotillomania. In this condition the self inflicted picking trauma is sufficient to cause appreciable damage to the nail and nail fold.

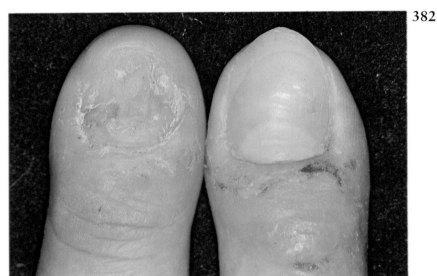
382

383 Onychotillomania: repeated pinching of the nails has caused subungual haemorrhages.

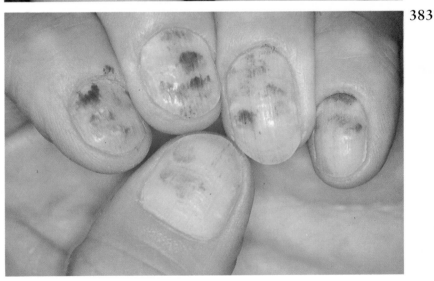
383

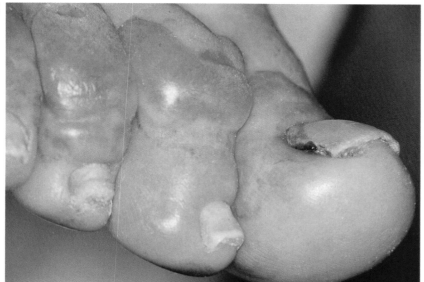

384 Rheumatoid-type arthritis. Periungual infarcts and haemorrhagic blisters occur as part of an associated cutaneous vasculitis (Bywaters syndrome).

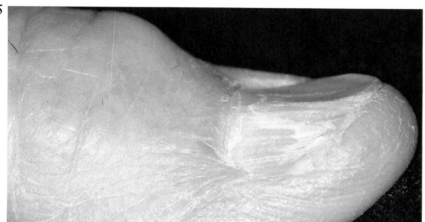

385 Rheumatoid arthritis: the nail is thinned and shows longitudinal ridging.

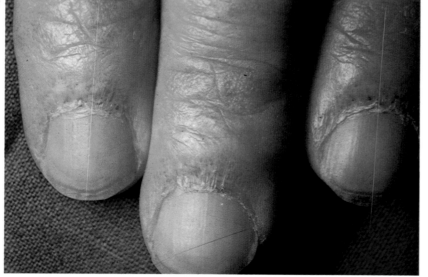

386 Dermatomyositis: the nail fold shows telangiectasia, thromboses, scarring and hyperkeratosis of the cuticle.

387 Dermatomyositis: early case showing erythema of the nail folds and red streaking along extensor tendons.

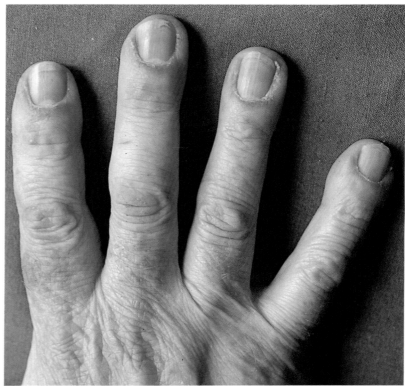

388 Systemic sclerosis, acrosclerosis. There is pallor and shrinkage of the finger pulps with beaking of the nails. (See also 365.)

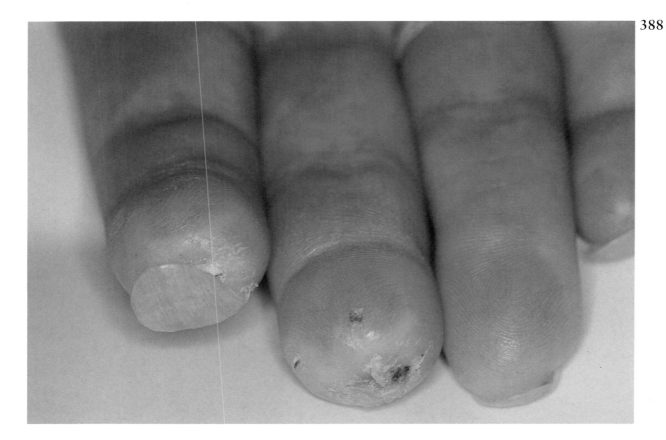

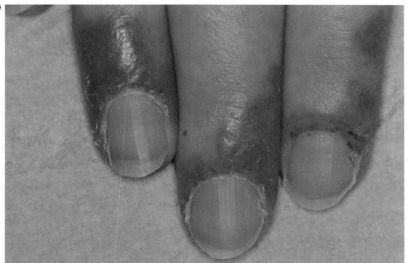

389 Systemic lupus erythematosus, chilblain type. Red plaques are seen around the nail folds.

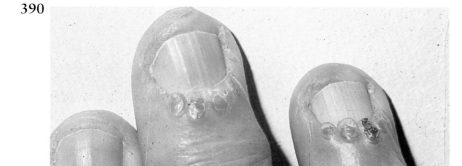

390 Multicentric reticulohistiocytosis. Red nodules, resmbling coral beads, are seen on the nail folds and digits; similar nodules are seen on the lips, nostrils and ears. There is often an associated severe arthritis mutilans. The condition affects mainly middle-aged women, about a quarter of whom are found to have a malignant neoplasm. (Courtesy Prof. H. Barriere.)

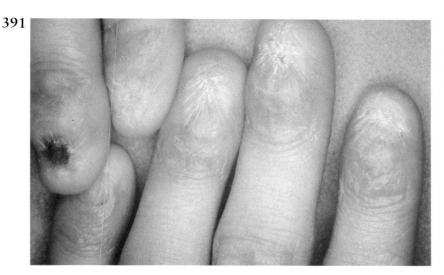

391 Graft versus host disease. Changes similar to those of lichen planus and scleroderma have been described, and pigmentation due to cytotoxic drugs may occur. (Courtesy Prof. J. Maleville.)

166

Nail changes in malignant disease

392 Clubbing in carcinoma of the bronchus. See also 259, 260.

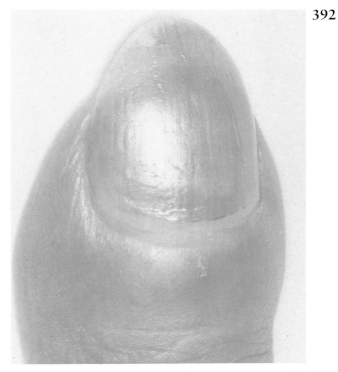

393 Glucagonoma syndrome is associated frequently, but not invariably, with carcinoma of the pancreas. In addition to the inflammation and fragmentation of the finger nails, there is necrolytic migratory erythema of the skin, and glossitis, anaemia and diabetes. (Courtesy Prof. J. Hewitt.)

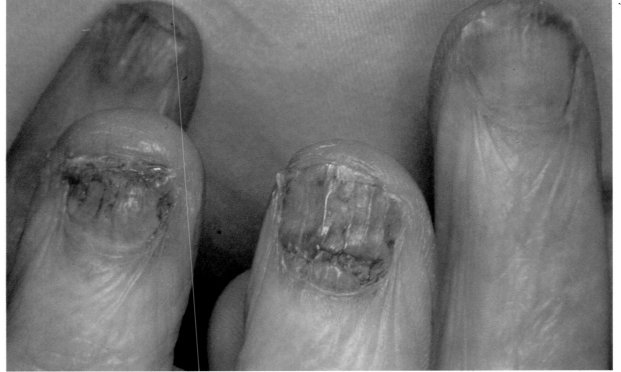

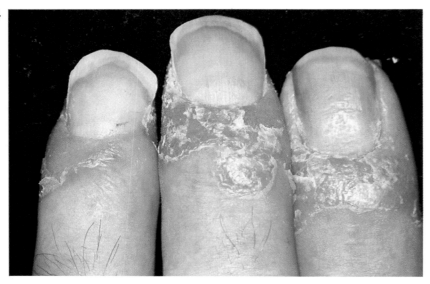

394 Acrokeratosis paraneoplastica (Bazex and Dupré). This condition affects mainly men over the age of 40. The psoriasiform changes of the extremities and nails are associated with malignant disease of the pharyngeal and laryngeal areas and the upper gastrointestinal and respiratory tracts.

Yellow nail syndrome: see 367. Occasionally carcinomas and lymphomas have been described as associated with this condition.

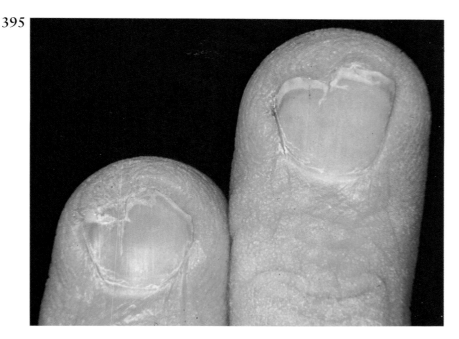

395 Acanthosis nigricans: warty hyperplasia of fingers and palms (tripe palms) is here associated with a distal nail dystrophy with vertical splitting of the nail. Acanthosis nigricans is associated with internal malignant disease. (Courtesy Dr. H. Baker.)

Drug eruptions and the nails

396 Antimalarial subungual pigmentation: a fairly common complication of continuous antimalarial therapy in tropical countries. The colour varies from shades of yellow and green to blue and blue-back. In quinacrine therapy, nail fluorescence under Wood's light is demonstrable even when the nails look otherwise normal.

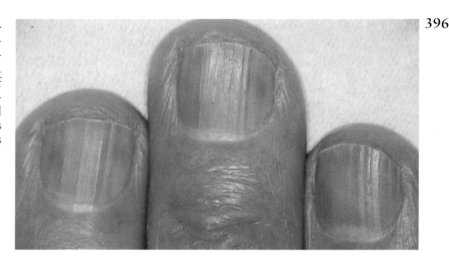

397 Photo-onycholysis. Photosensitivity is associated with onycholysis and dyschromia. The nails are often tender at the time of the onset of the problem. The compounds most commonly responsible are demethyl-chlortetracycline and doxycycline.

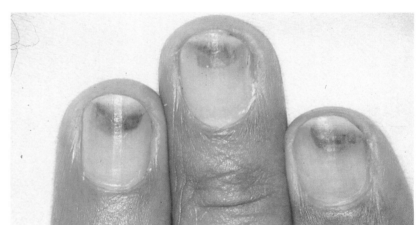

398 Psoralens, subungual haemorrhage. Photo-onycholysis together with subungual haemorrhage (shown here) is seen when psoralens are used systemically as part of photochemotherapy (PUVA). Irregular and banded brown nail pigmentation may rarely occur. (Courtesy Dr. C. Grupper.)

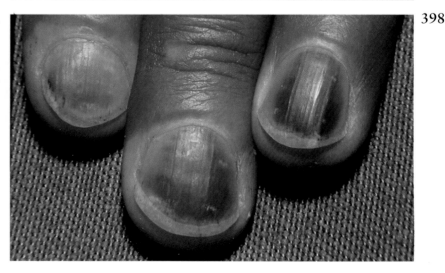

399

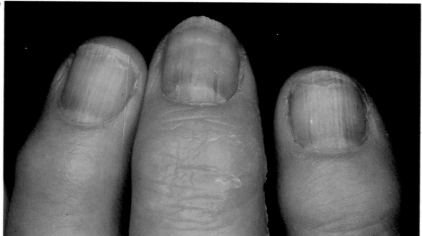

399 Argyria: blue nails, generally restricted to the lunular region, are part of systemic argyria. Similar changes, due to a defect in copper metabolism, are seen in Wilson's disease. (Courtesy Prof. J. Mascaro.)

400

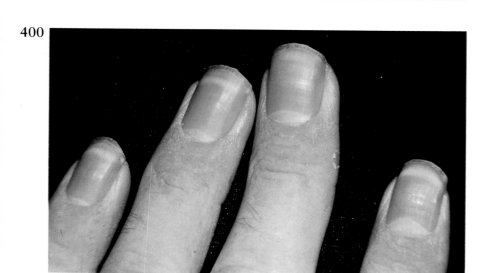

400 Acute arsenical poisoning: Mees' lines. These are white transverse striations, usually single, that can be shown on analysis to contain arsenic. This is important for medico-legal reasons. (Courtesy Prof. J. Mascaro.)

401

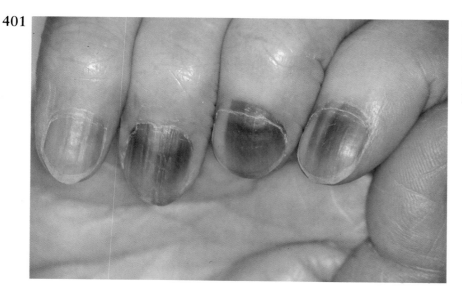

401 Cytotoxic drugs: pigmentation due to a drug given for leukaemia. Particularly found after treatment with doxyrubicin, busulphan and cyclophosphamide.

402 Cytotoxic drugs: prominent transverse white bands were seen following intermittent therapy with the drug. (Courtesy Dr. M. Jeanmougin and Prof. J. Civatte.)

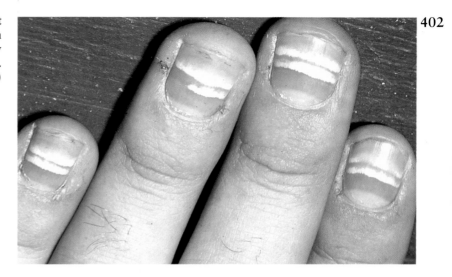

403 Retinoids: oral retinoids can cause thinning of nails and nail folds changes of paronychia and granulation tissue that develop in the lateral nail grooves and may be associated with fragility.

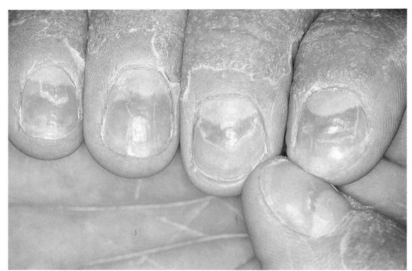

404 Pyogenic granuloma due to oral retinoid drug. (Courtesy Dr. J. Delescluse.)

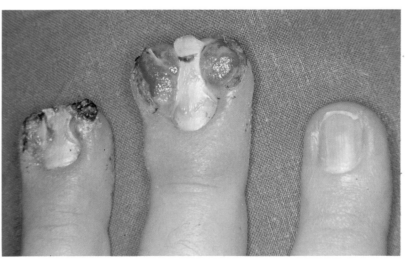

Occupation-related nail disorders

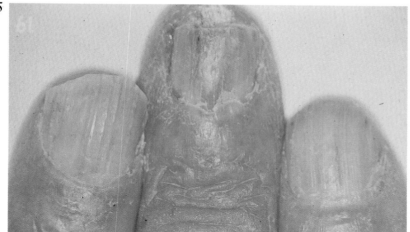

405 Radiodermatitis. There are changes of ridging and fragility of the nail plate with redness, atrophy and keratosis of the surrounding nail folds, which may present with paronychia. The condition has been seen in dentists who take their own X-rays and physicians who have consistently practised X-ray screening without protective gloves.

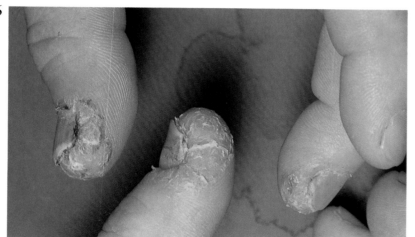

406 Tulip finger: dermatitis and hyperkeratosis arising from allergic contact dermatitis brought about by contact with a constituent of the tulip bulb. The condition starts under the free margin of the nail and spreads to the finger tips and periungual regions.

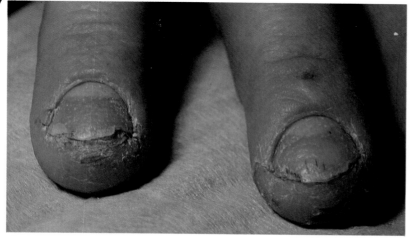

407 Epoxy resin dermatitis: the resin oligomer may collect under the free edge of the nail and polymerize slowly as it dries. The changes affect the finger tip, the distal subungual area and the lateral nail folds. There is often associated allergic contact dermatitis elsewhere on the skin.

408 Hairdresser's nail changes. Hairdressers are liable to occupational chronic paronychia and onycholysis with embedding of hairs into the nail folds and subungual tissue.

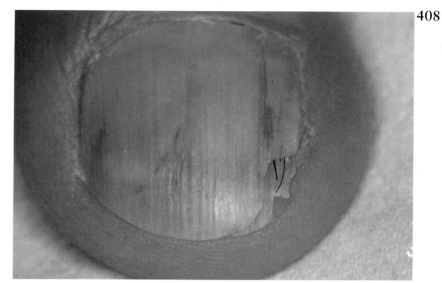

409 Pesticide nail changes. Insecticides and weed killers can produce pigmentary abnormalities and softening of the nail plate. This example shows a yellowish-white appearance of the proximal part of the nails due to dinitro-orthocresol.

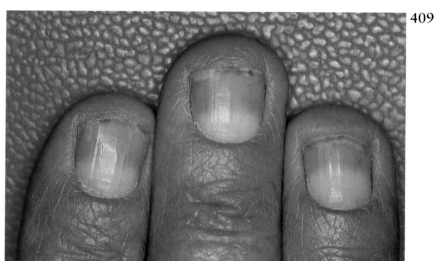

410 Photographer's nails: this appearance resulted from use of a developer, metol. The arcuate pattern of the proximal part of the staining indicates that it is exogenous.

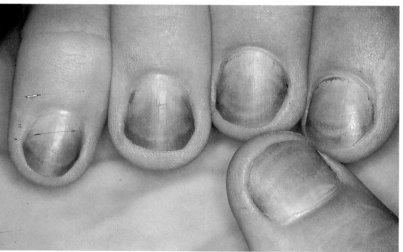

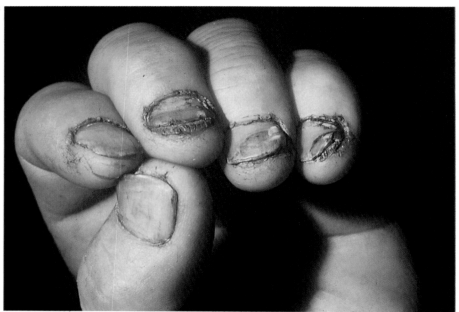

411 Worn down nails: koilonychia with onycholysis and wearing down of the lateral sides of the nails. This appearance can arise from heavy manual occupations such as handling heavy bulky bags or sacks. (Courtesy Dr. B. Schubert.)

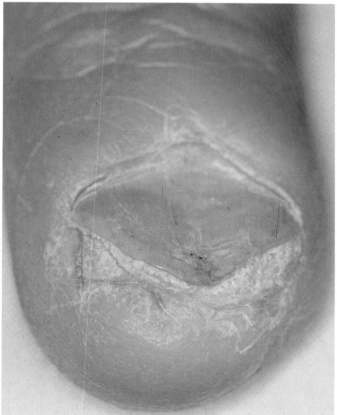

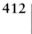

412 Worn down nail, showing lateral hyperkeratosis.

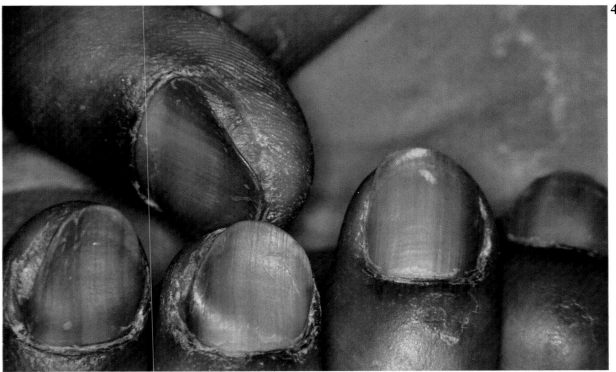

413 Worn down nails. This patient shows koilonychia, lateral onycholysis and subungual hyperkeratosis affecting the thumb, index and middle finger nails. This pattern is common in occupational koilonychia.

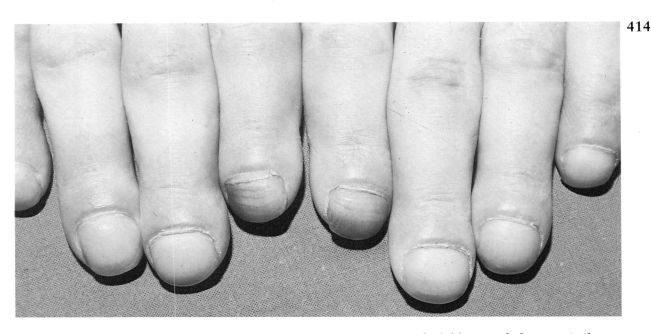

414 Acro-osteolysis in PVC (polyvinylchloride) disease: there is pseudoclubbing and changes similar to those seen in systemic sclerosis. The condition occurs in individuals involved in the making of PVC, but the disorder has been associated with inhalation of the monomer, monovinylchloride. (Courtesy Prof. G. Moulin.)

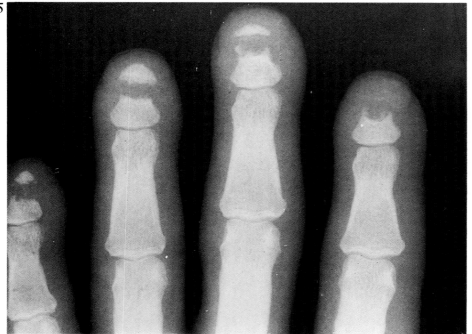

415 Acro-osteolysis in PVC disease: X-ray. The bony defect in the distal phalanges is well shown. (Courtesy Prof. G. Moulin.)

Cosmetic-associated disorders

416 Nail varnish staining. Orange staining of the distal two-thirds of the nail plate occurs in relatively few individuals who use nail varnish.

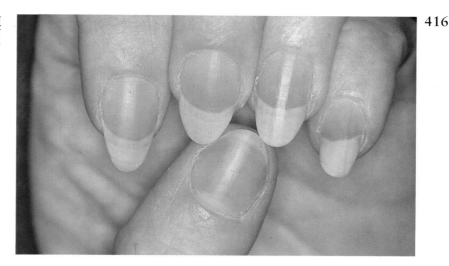

417 Nail hardener changes: onycholysis and painful subungual haematomas can follow repeated application of formaldehyde nail hardeners.

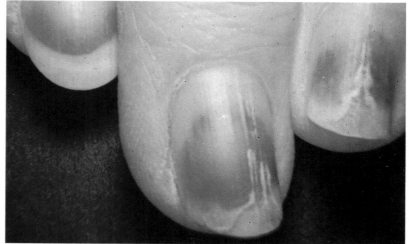

418 Sculptured nails. In this technique an acrylic mixture is used to create a new nail *in situ*, using a template. This can be followed by allergic contact dermatitis of the periungual skin, with onycholysis, and even distant contact dermatitis (especially of the face). Sometimes there is persistent paraesthesiae of the finger tips, a condition also found in orthopaedic surgeons who use acrylic resins.

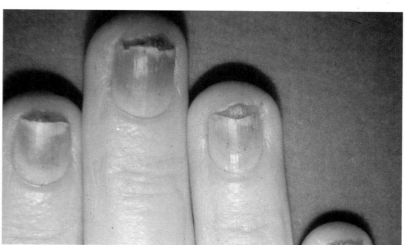

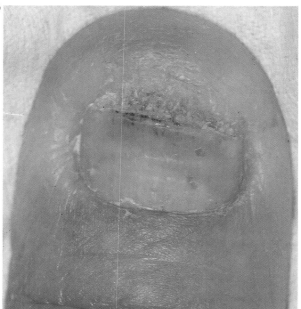

419 Artificial nail effects. Preformed plastic nail prostheses are kept in place with a variety of glues and resins. In this patient there has been almost complete cessation of growth with distal hyperkeratosis of the nail bed lasting for several months.

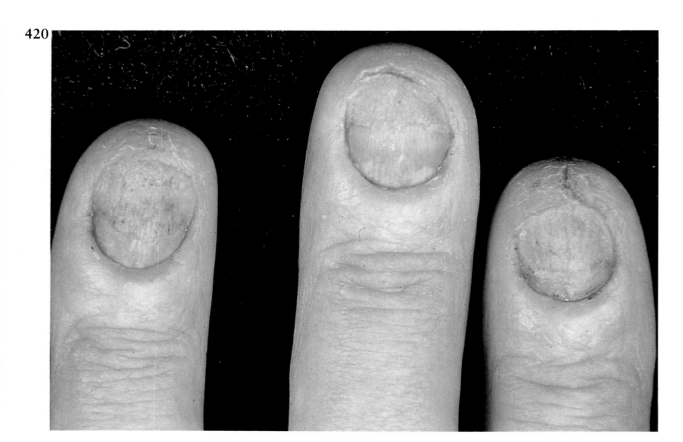

420 Nail atrophy: an example of subungual hyperkeratosis and onycholysis, with finger tip dryness and fissuring. It was due to paratertiary butyl phenol formaldehyde resin, traced to a particular batch of adhesive used to attach a brand of plastic artificial nail.

Genetic nail disorders

421 Anonychia: congenital absence of nail found in a patient with ectodermal dysplasia.

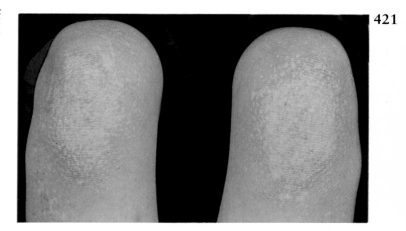

421

422 Pachyonychia congenita: the nail beds are thickened, discoloured and extremely hard. The combination of thickening and hypercurvature gives a barrel shape to the nails.

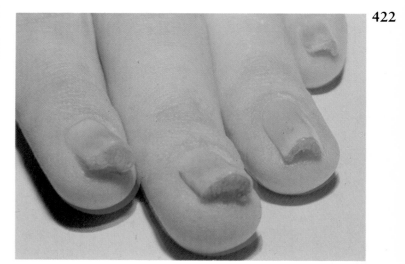

422

423 Pachyonychia congenita: a lateral view showing a nail resembling a horse's hoof.

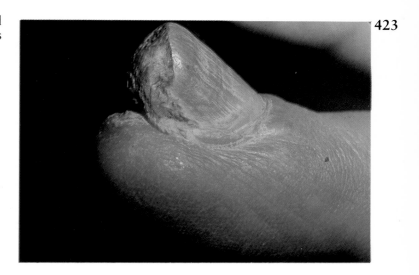

423

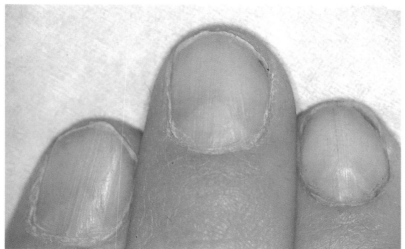

424 Nail–patella syndrome. The characteristic nail changes are triangular lunulae (shown here) and partial absence of thumb nails.

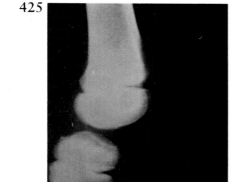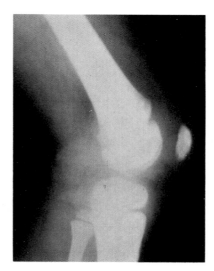

425 Nail–patella syndrome: X-ray. The absence of patella is demonstrated in the lateral knee X-ray on the left. A normal knee X-ray is shown for comparison on the right. A pathognomonic radiological sign is the presence of iliac crest horns seen on pelvic X-rays.

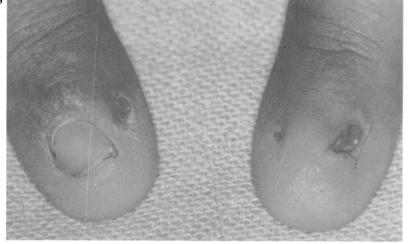

426 Congenital onychodysplasia of the index fingers (COIF syndrome, Iso–Kikuchi syndrome). Micronychia and polyonychia are seen in the finger on the left, and rudimentary polyonychia is shown in the finger on the right. Other digits may be affected. (Courtesy Prof. A. Claudy.)

427 Epidermolysis bullosa dystrophica. Nail changes are common in several varieties of epidermolysis bullosa, secondary to blistering. Nails tend to be present in dominantly inherited varieties and absent in recessive forms. (Courtesy Prof. P. Lauret.)

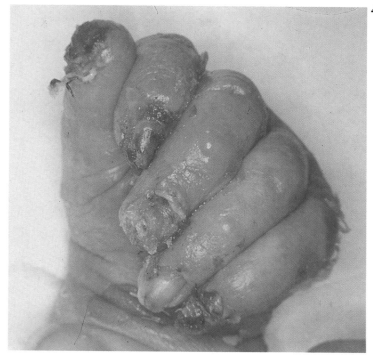

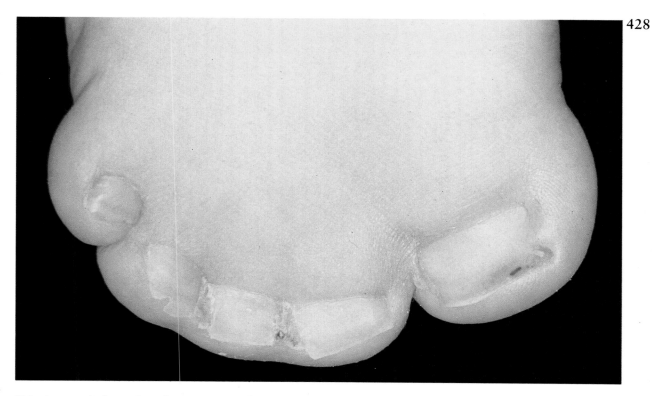

428 Acrocephalosyndactyly (Apert's syndrome): a foot showing marked syndactyly due to anomalies of the bony phalanges. The nails are broad. Various other skeletal abnormalities are found.

Tumours of the nail apparatus

A large variety of tumours can occur in association with the nails. A selection of the commoner and more important ones is illustrated.

429

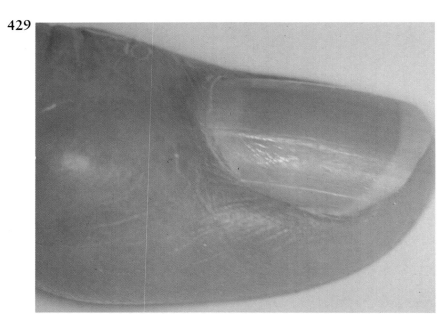

429 Myxoid cyst: here affecting the nail matrix leading to a wide longitudinal groove in the nail plate.

430

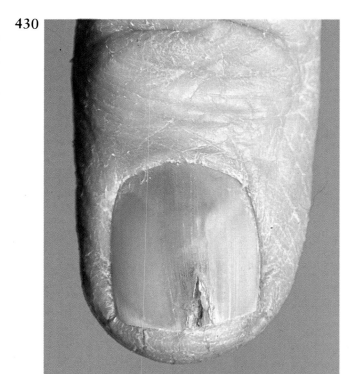

430 Glomus tumour, subungual: a red spot is seen in the lunular region with splitting of the free edge of the nail. It was extremely tender on pressure.

431 Pyogenic granuloma of the finger tip. These lesions bleed easily and are usually secondary to minor trauma. The specimen should always be sent to histopathology to rule out an amelanotic melanoma.

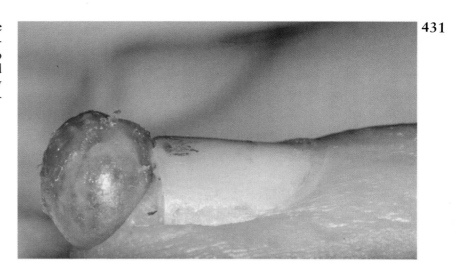

432 Subungual exostosis. There is only slight onycholysis; the main symptom was tenderness.

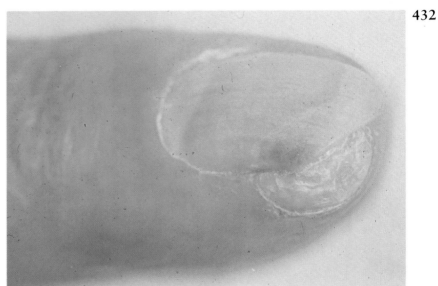

433 Subungual exostosis: X-ray. The same patient as in **432**. The exostosis is seen arising from the dorsal aspect of the distal bony phalanx.

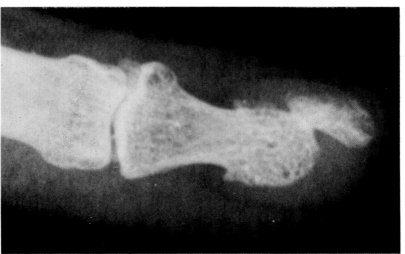

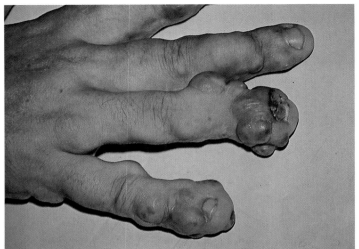

434 Maffucci's syndrome. Failure of normal ossification leads to subcutaneous tumorous masses of cartilage and haemangiomas. Deformity or loss of the nails occurs when the distal phalanges are affected.

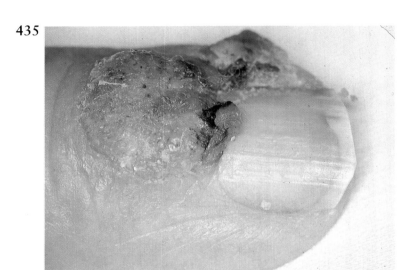

435 Bowen's disease: shown here is the warty hyperkeratotic variety of the disorder, involving the proximal nail fold, extending to one lateral nail fold. The differential diagnosis from viral wart and squamous carcinoma is made by histology.

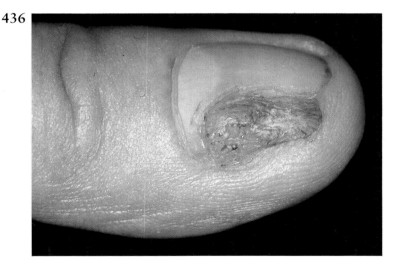

436 Squamous cell carcinoma: partial progressive destruction of the nail plate from the tumour that is arising in the nail bed. Biopsy is essential.

437 Longitudinal melanonychia. The problem in this condition is the diagnosis of the cause: medical, e.g. Addison's disease, cytotoxic drugs etc.; or surgical, or dermatological, e.g. melanocytic naevus or malignant melanoma. While such bands are often physiological in black people, in Caucasians biopsy is often required to establish the cause.

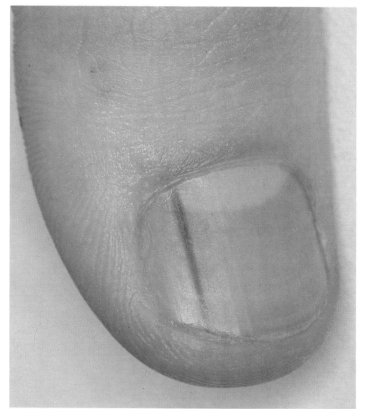

438 Longitudinal melanonychia: same patient as in **437**. The nail fold has been retracted surgically to reveal the origin of the band, which is the site from which the biopsy should be taken.

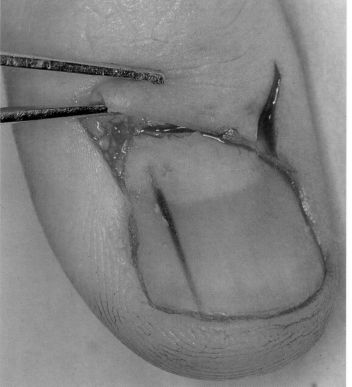

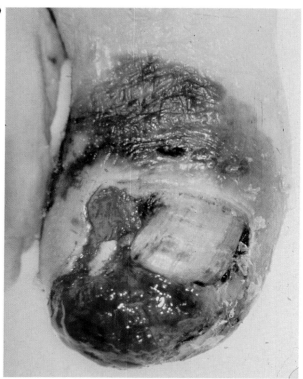 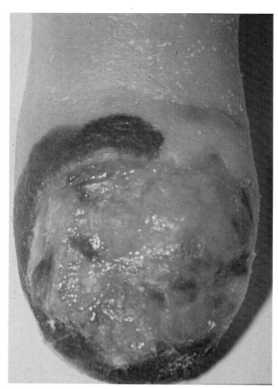

439, 440 Malignant melanoma. The digit shown on the left shows partial destruction of the nail plate, whereas the one on the right has lost its nail plate completely. Both show the pathognomonic feature of spreading pigmentation (Hutchinson's sign).

441 Malignant melanoma: a type with wide linear melanonychia; negroid subject.

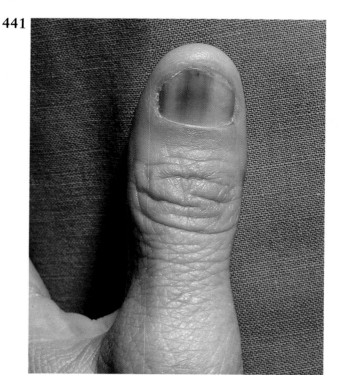

442 Amelanotic melanoma. There is loss of the central portion of the nail plate due to the growth of tissue resembling pyogenic granuloma, which is in fact malignant melanoma. Biopsy is crucial.

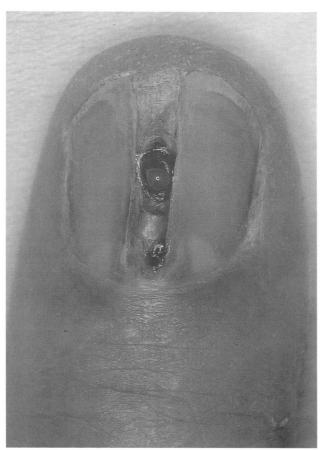

Index

Figures in bold *type refer to figure numbers, those in light type are page numbers*

Traction alopecia **96**
Traumatic alopecia 49–52, 95–106
Trichofolliculoma 89, **236**
Trichomycosis axillaris 65, **156–8**
Trichonodosis 39, **87–8**
Trichophyton
–*mentagrophytes* 65, **146**
–*mentagrophytes* var. *interdigitale* 322
–*quinckeanum* **146**
–*rubrum* **146**, 318, 325
–*schoenleinii* 65, **148**
–*verrucosum* 65, **144**, **146**
Trichoptilosis 39
Trichorrhexis invaginata **72**
Trichorrhexis nodosa **13–14**, 39
Trichostasis spinulosa 39
Trichotillomania 37, 49, **98–104**
Tripe palms **395**
Trumpet nail **265**
Tulip finger **406**
Turban tumour 89, **219**
Twenty nail dystrophy **315**

Uncombable hair syndrome (*cheveux incoiffables*) 39, **83–5**

Varicella 73
Viral warts 65, **160**, **333–4**
Vitiligo 62, **139–41**

Washboard thumb nails **286**, **381**
Weathering of hair 17, **13–17**, **22–3**, 39
White bands **369**, **402**
White nails 126, 322, 371
–*see also* Leukonychia
Whitlow, herpetic **331**
Wilson's disease **399**
Wood's light 65
Woolly hair 39, **79–80**
Woolly naevus 39, **81–2**
Worn down nails 271, **411–13**

X-ray alopecia **132–3**
X-ray damaged skin **255**
Xanthoma 89, **231**

Yellow nail syndrome 125, 126, 367, 168

Zinc deficiency 73, **168–9**, 308